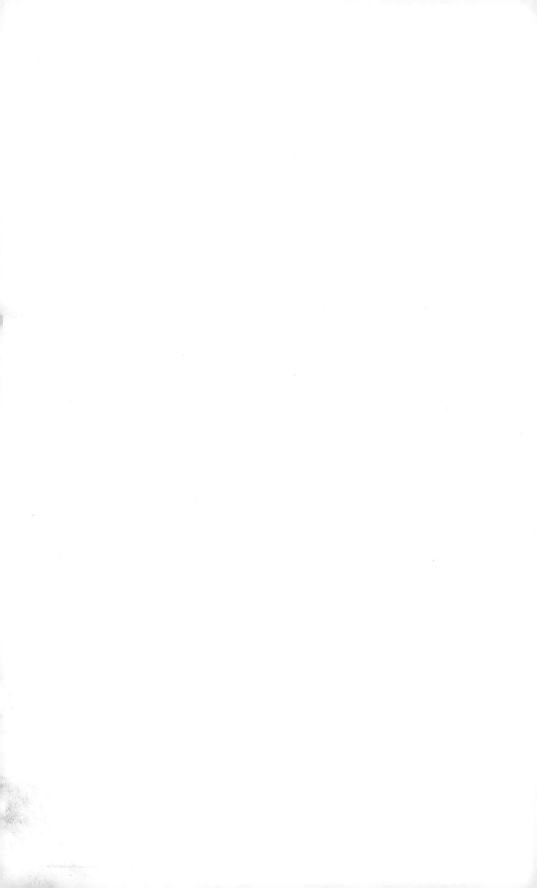

Detection of Malingering during Head Injury Litigation

Arthur MacNeill Horton, Jr. • Cecil R. Reynolds
Editors

Detection of Malingering during Head Injury Litigation

Third Edition

Volume 1

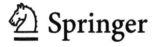 Springer

Editors
Arthur MacNeill Horton, Jr.
Neuropsychology Section
Psych Associates of Maryland
Towson and Columbia
Bethesda, MD, USA

Cecil R. Reynolds
Department of Educational Psychology
Texas A&M University College Station
Austin, TX, USA

ISBN 978-3-030-54655-7   ISBN 978-3-030-54656-4   (eBook)
https://doi.org/10.1007/978-3-030-54656-4

This Springer imprint is published by the registered company Springer Nature Switzerland AG
The registered company address is: Gewerbestrasse 11, 6330 Cham, Switzerland

Preface

The issue of potential malingering (or poor effort) in the context of head injury litigation has seen an explosion of research and commentary in the last 40 years. Various journals devoted to clinical neuropsychology practice of the 1950s, 1960s, and 1970s rarely published papers focused on the issue of malingering in civil litigation. The few papers that were published deal with malingering in regard to military service and criminal prosecution. It might be recalled that clinical neuropsychology began as an academic research endeavor.

Only after empirical studies proved the validity of neuropsychological evaluations as measures of brain behavior relationships was the necessary basis of scientific findings to support clinical applications established. Ralph Reitan, Oscar Parsons, Arthur Benton, and a bevy of their former students (Lawrence Hartlage and Charles Mathews, among others) published empirical research studies demonstrating the importance of clinical neuropsychology research to patient care. Their work formed the basis for clinical practice in neuropsychology. An interesting clinical note is that Dr. Benton initially developed his famous Visual Retention Test based on his clinical work during World War II, when Dr. Benton was based at the San Diego Veterans Administration Hospital and had to assess possible malingering by sailors who did not wish to return to fighting in the Pacific.

This growth of clinical neuropsychology research, clinical practitioners, and concurrent founding of journals to support scholarly inquiry and clinical practice has produced many revelations about the effects of closed head injury, an injury which was for many years believed to be of little consequence and one known as a silent epidemic. Coupled with the explosive growth of knowledge about the potential deleterious effects of closed head injury there has been increased personal injury litigation, changes in protocols for screening, assessment, and treatment of sports-related and war-related head injuries, and product liability suits. As more and more head injuries have come to be litigated and the potential sums of money involved have become enormous, issues and concerns about malingering (or poor effort) have grown substantially. By the 1980s, detection of malingering and its evaluation had found a routine place in the primary journals of neuropsychology.

The first edition of this book attempted to address the problem of malingering in head injury litigation. Several things were clear at the time of the first edition. The first was that malingering was a very substantial problem in head injury litigation. For example, empirical research findings had indicated that at least 25% of cases of head injury in litigation involve malingering. Second, the possibility of malingering existed in all head injury litigation cases and clinicians needed to be prepared to make the diagnosis when it was the most probable diagnosis. Third, there were many methodological, conceptual, and logistical caveats related to the detection of malingering. Fourth, there are emotional difficulties in labeling a patient a malingerer.

Malingering is a diagnosis with clear negative implications and is tantamount to calling a potentially brain injured patient a liar, something that can have very negative personal and financial consequences. Because of the very serious consequences, very convincing evidence is required for such a diagnosis and more than is the case for many clinical diagnoses made on a routine basis. The first edition attempted to demonstrate the utility and the pitfalls of various actuarial and clinical approaches to the diagnosis of malingering and equip the clinician with the necessary tools, knowledge, and logic to consider malingering and its alternative diagnoses intelligently, honestly, and ethically.

In the years that have passed since the first edition was published, much had happened in terms of research and clinical practice related to the detection of malingering in head injury litigation. For example, a new common practice was to use preferentially the term "poor effort" rather than "malingering," as poor effort is a behavior that can be observed objectively. Research has shown in adults that effort explained 50% of the variance in the whole neuropsychological test battery but years of education explained only 12%, and severity of brain injury and age explained 4% and 3% respectively (Green, Rohling, Lees-Haley, & Allen, 2001). Also in children Kirkwood, Yeates, Randolph, and Kirk (2011) found while failure rates on effort tests were lower in children than in adults, effort testing explained 38% of the variance in the neuropsychological test battery.

On the other hand, the term malingering has been thought to require the forming of a conscious intention which as yet is unobservable in addition to a behavior. While it is clear that in the future it may be possible to determine if an individual has formed an intention to malinger as of the time, it has not been scientifically established. With the above concern noted, the term malingering is used in the title of this volume but the editors are aware of its limitations.

In the second edition of this work, the assembled chapters were based on rigorous scientific research but were also clinically oriented to facilitate their application to practice. Opening chapters disclosed the methodological and conceptual problems in the diagnosis of malingering to establish a clear mind-set of critical analysis before reading about methods proposed by other authors. The chapters that followed provided then current methods and thinking on multiple approaches to the detection of malingering during head injury litigation, including specific symptoms such as memory loss to more global claims of diffuse loss of function to cognitive and psychomotor arenas. The various presentations ranged from the strong actuarial methods to careful, consummate clinical reasoning. The second edition, similar to the first edition, had been developed for the thoughtful, serious clinician who may be involved in evaluating patients with head injury who often become involved in litigation with regard to these injuries.

In the years since the second edition was published, there has been considerable additional research regarding malingering. A major conceptual change has been the distinction between performance validity and symptom validity. Briefly performance validity refers to malingering or effort tests that assess physical performance, be it motor or verbal. For example, the Word Memory Test (WMT) or Test of Malingered Memory (TOMM) would be examples of performance validity tests. In contrast, symptom validity refers to self-report that may be false for the purpose of feigning. The classic example of a symptom validity test is the various validity scales on the Minnesota Multiphasic Personality Inventory (MMPI) (in various editions such as the MMPI-2, MMPI-2-RF, and MMPI-3).

In addition, recent years have shown a great explosion in tests of effort using patterns of performance and cutting scores on neuropsychological tests not initially designed to assess effort to assess effort. Moreover, the large volume of clinical research has prompted many strong ideas and creative approaches and new methodologies to the detection of malingering. Due to the efforts of multiple researchers the diagnosis of malingering has profited from the establishment of a greater empirical scientific basis for decision-making.

The diagnosis of malingering is still, however, fraught with conceptual, philosophical, and logistical potholes. Because much has happened in the research basis for this clinical and forensic area, it is felt that a new third edition is required to address new research findings and changes in clinical practice that have occurred since the publishing of the second edition of this book.

This new third edition is intended to address new research findings and changes in clinical practice that have occurred since the publishing of the second edition of this book and provide practitioners with the necessary contemporary scientific findings to guide their clinical work and ensure that their patients receive the highest quality of clinical neuropsychological services.

Because of the increase in new research, it was decided to enlarge the third edition into two volumes. In the first volume, the authors (Faust, Gaudet, Ahern, and Bridges) discuss the complex methodological and conceptual problems in the diagnosis of malingering to clearly establish a mind-set of critical analysis before reading about issues and methods proposed by other authors. In the second volume, the authors address ethical issues (Kaufman and Bush), cultural aspects (Braw), and neuroimaging (Bigler). Specific test focused research is provided in chapters that follow related to the Word Memory Test (WMT), Medical Symptom Validity Test (MSVT) and Nonverbal-Medical Symptom Validity Test (NV-MSVT) (Armistead-Jehle, Denney, and Shura), Test of Malingered Memory (TOMM) (Perna), executive functioning tests (Suhr, Bryant, and Cook), and the MMPI-2, MMPI-2-RF, and MMPI-3 (Tylicki, Tarescavage, and Wygant). The next chapter is focused on assessing malingering in pediatric evaluations (Clegg, Lynch, Mian, and McCaffrey). The last chapter focuses on methods and techniques for applying the information in the earlier chapters in forensic litigation (McCaffrey, Mian, Clegg, and Lynch).

The editors must express their appreciation to the chapter authors, who have made important contributions to the evaluation of malingering (or poor effort). Each has provided original insights, methods, and commentary on these very complex and difficult issues. Their willingness to share in the movement toward advancement in the diagnosis of malingering is greatly appreciated. To our editor at Springer, we would like to express our appreciation for the continuing faith in our efforts to produce a work that contributes significantly to the growth of clinical neuropsychology and the appropriate diagnosis of malingering (or poor effort). To the Springer staff and production editor, we also thank you for bringing the manuscript to its published conclusion with such promptness. To our two long-suffering wives, Mary W. Horton and Dr. Julia A. Hickman, goes our continuing and unfaltering love and appreciation for their help, support, kindness, and understanding during those times devoted to manuscripts such as this that pull from time otherwise spent together. We love you and thank you; we thank you very much!

Bethesda, MD, USA   Arthur MacNeill Horton
Austin, TX, USA   Cecil R. Reynolds

Conflicts of Interest Dr. Horton was a test consultant for the development of the Pediatric Performance Validity Test Suite (PdPVTS) and revision of the Test of Memory Malingering (TOMM) and received honoraria for his service but does not receive income from sales of the PdPVTS or the revised TOMM.

Dr. Reynolds is an author of the PdPVTS along with numerous other psychological and neuropsychological tests and receives royalties from their sales.

References

Green, P., Rohling, M. L., Lees-Haley, P. R., & Allen, L. M. (2001). Effort has a greater effect on test scores than severe brain injury in compensation claimants. *Brain Injury, 15*(12), 1045–1060.

Kirkwood, M. W., Yeates, K. O., Randolph, C., & Kirk, J. W. (2011). The implications of symptom validity test failure for ability-based test performance in a pediatric sample. *Psychological Assessment, 24*(1), 36–45. https://doi.org/10.1037/a0024628.

Contents

Assessment of Malingering and Falsification: Continuing to Push the Boundaries of Knowledge in Research and Clinical Practice

David F. Faust, Charles E. Gaudet, David C. Ahern, and Ana J. Bridges

How can one make both a false-negative and a valid-positive identification simultaneously? Co-occurring correct and incorrect judgments can result either by identifying an injured individual who is also exaggerating deficit simply as a malingerer, or by identifying that same individual only as injured. In the first instance one misses the injury while correctly identifying malingering, and in the second instance one correctly identifies the injury but misses malingering.

As this example illustrates, the assessment of falsification or malingering often does not fall into neat packages. Impressive advances have led to the development of better methods, better strategies, broader options, enhanced awareness, and greater understanding, with psychologists and neuropsychologists easily being the most productive contributors to these noteworthy developments. However, critical problems and diagnostic puzzles remain, and as is often true as science advances, those problems tend to be considerably deeper and more complex than might first be realized. There is still a great deal more to learn about this domain, and in this volume we try to contribute in some small way to this endeavor. Ultimately,

D. F. Faust (✉)
Department of Psychology, University of Rhode Island and Department of Psychiatry and Human Behavior, Alpert Medical School of Brown University, Kingston, RI, USA
e-mail: faust@uri.edu

C. E. Gaudet
Department of Psychology, University of Rhode Island, Kingston, RI, USA

Psychology Service, VA Boston Healthcare System, Boston, MA, USA

Department of Psychiatry, Harvard Medical School, Boston, MA, USA

D. C. Aher1n
Department of Psychiatry & Human Behavior, Alpert Medical School of Brown University, Providence, RI, USA

A. J. Bridges
Department of Psychological Science, University of Arkansas, Fayetteville, AR, USA

© Springer Nature Switzerland AG 2021
A. M. Horton, Jr., C. R. Reynolds (eds.), *Detection of Malingering during Head Injury Litigation*, https://doi.org/10.1007/978-3-030-54656-4_1

1

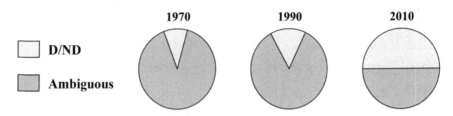

Fig. 1 Progress in increasing the proportion of Definitive or Near-Definitive (D/ND) cases

improved understanding and methods serve equally to identify false claims and verify true ones, and thus enhance the capacity of our profession to assist in such important tasks as the just resolution of legal conflicts, which is the normative role for expert witnesses.

One way to represent scientific progress is to divide pertinent cases into those that can be identified with certainty or near certainty versus those that remain ambiguous or difficult to identify and to look at changes in the proportions of these categories over time. We will refer to the former type of case as D/ND (definitive or near-definitive) and the latter as AMB (ambiguous). Of course, we are dichotomizing matters that lie on a continuum, but for current purposes finer divisions or more precise boundaries are not required because the intent is mainly conceptual. As shown in Fig. 1, suppose we traced the distribution of cases over the last 4 decades as follows, while presuming the level of ambiguous cases continues to gradually decline as of today.

We do not wish to debate the specific divisions across the pie charts for the moment. Given the accuracy rates that many studies yield, a reader might reject the proportions in the pie charts as misleadingly low, especially in the chart for 2010. We are not claiming that the proportions should be taken literally, the intent here being to illustrate progress over time. With that said, for reasons we will later address extensively, the results of many research studies, although certainly positive and encouraging, may substantially overestimate accuracy rates. In particular, many such studies primarily involve relatively clear or extreme cases as opposed to more ambiguous or difficult cases. Whatever one's position on these matters, we believe there would be broad consensus about the positive trends represented in the successive charts and the expectation that further gains have been made post-2010 and continuing to the present time.

As scientific knowledge has advanced, the percentage of cases that can be identified with high levels of accuracy has increased, with particular acceleration in progress during the last few decades as the level and quality of research have shown remarkable growth. The more we can whittle away at the remaining ambiguous cases (whatever their estimated frequency might be), the better off we will be, and it is sensible to focus research efforts on the types of cases that, despite our efforts so far, remain ambiguous or difficult. We might anticipate that these sorts of cases can present considerable scientific challenges, for if they were easy we would already know how to identify them. In many domains (e.g., golf, budget cutting, work efficiency), further advances can become progressively more difficult for various reasons, in particular because one can start with components that are easier to correct and because initial low levels of proficiency leave greater room and opportunity for gain. Without losing sight of the impressive strides that have been made, the main focus of this volume is on these remaining ambiguous cases, not because we wish to concentrate on the negative but because they are a key to advancing proficiency—to achieving positive gains. Such cases often create significant scientific challenges and will require concentrated effort at least comparable to that which has already been expended. However, we think the prospects for further advance are good and that the effort is well justified given the importance of the problem.

Two areas of focus are critical to advance, and discussing them briefly at this juncture should provide a flavor for the sorts of matters we will cover. One is increased study of an underrepresented yet common group in litigation—those who are brain injured *and* falsifying. (Researchers studying psychological disorders have been giving more attention to co-presenting conditions for a number of years now, despite the challenges involved, and we believe it would be wise to do so for co-occurrences or co-phenomena in the area of falsification and malingering as well.) Unless one takes the extremist view that any and all falsification renders a person undeserving of any compensation (i.e., that the deserved retribution or consequence is the complete negation of any meritorious claims), a position we believe holds individuals to a standard of near-infallibility or moral perfection, then this group deserves our attention. Whatever our personal views on the matter, the outcome that should result when there is both legitimate injury and falsification has occupied and will occupy the trier of fact daily in courtrooms across the country, and it is an area in which mental health professionals could play a very important role in fostering more informed decisions, if and when sufficient research progress is made.

Second, our seemingly bright prospects for scientific advance in the appraisal of falsification hinges to no small extent on recognizing and correcting what we call the *extreme group problem* in research. Much contemporary research may not go far in reducing the percentage of ambiguous cases and may even produce the opposite result (i.e., lead us to miss cases we might identify correctly otherwise). These negative consequences stem largely from sampling problems in research, which result in groups that differ quantitatively and qualitatively from the remaining ambiguous cases. As we will argue, the extreme group problem is a common, highly impactful, yet often subtle methodological flaw. It is especially pernicious because the extent of the flaw may often be the most powerful influence on the accuracy rates obtained in studies, that is, the worse the flaw, the better a method seems to perform. When there is a powerful (or predominant) *positive* association between the magnitude of a design flaw and obtained accuracy rates, and this flaw goes unrecognized, a multitude of serious negative consequences are likely to follow. We will describe how the extreme group problem can be parsed and possibly corrected, although it may require substantial conceptual reframing, new avenues of research, and new metrics to detect, measure, and attenuate or negate its effects.

Our aim is not to critique the now considerable body of literature study-by-study, nor to address fundamental methodological points that have been cogently and convincingly described in the literature. Rather, our main intent is conceptual and prospective, with a particular focus on critical problems that may be under-recognized and suggestions and strategies that may assist in tackling challenging methodological hurdles.

1   Limitations of Experience in Learning to Detect Malingering: Benefits of Augmenting Clinical Judgment with Formal Methods

The intensity of reaction sometimes seen when research has raised questions about clinicians' capacity to detect malingering, especially absent the use of specialized methods and when depending primarily on subjective or professional judgment, seems to have quieted down as mounting scientific studies have made matters increasingly clear. Even more than 20 years ago, based on the additional evidence collected by that time, Williams (1998) put the matter thusly:

> The study of malingering has moved beyond the controversies about whether clinicians are able and willing to detect it… the developing literature clearly suggests that clinicians using conventional strategies of interpretation cannot detect malingering and need some new systematic approach to the interpretation of conventional tests or new specialized symptom validity tests. (p. 126)

Although one might have preferred a different descriptor than "cannot detect malingering" such as "may have considerable difficulty" or "are highly prone to error," the same basic conclusions are echoed in more tempered form in the National Academy of Neuropsychology's position paper on malingering detection (Bush et al., 2005) and the American Academy of Clinical Neuropsychology's publication on this same topic (Heilbronner, Sweet, Morgan, Larrabee, & Millis, 2009). In these sources one will find statements such as "[U]se of psychometric indicators is the most valid approach to identifying neuropsychological response validity" (Heilbronner et al., 2009, p. 1106) and "[S]ubjective indicators, such as examinee statements and examiner observations, should be afforded less weight due to the lack of scientific evidence supporting their validity" (Bush et al., 2005, p. 424). Research supporting such statements includes studies demonstrating the difficulty of detecting lies or misrepresentations, the limits of experience and clinical judgment in learning to detect and identify malingering, and the potential and sometimes sizeable benefits realized when specialized methods are applied meticulously and interpreted in strict accord with scientifically based, formal decision procedures (see Faust, 2011, Chaps. 8 and 17).

Nevertheless, experience often has a powerful pull on clinical judgment and decision making. Given the inflated impression of efficacy that can easily result from experientially based impressions and its potential *detrimental* effects on accuracy in malingering detection when it overrides the use of more effective methods, the limitations of learning via experience in this domain are worth examining. One can start by considering the conditions that promote or inhibit experiential learning (Dawes, 1989; Faust, 1989; Faust & Faust, 2011). Experiential learning tends to be most successful when feedback is immediate, clear, and deterministic. By *deterministic*, we mean that the feedback is unfailingly or perfectly related to its antecedent, in particular the accuracy of judgments or conclusions. Thus, each time we are right we find out we are right, and each time we are wrong we are informed so. At the other end of the spectrum, learning can be difficult or impossible when no feedback is received. In between, as the error term in feedback increases, that is, as the level of noise and inaccuracy in feedback grows, the more difficult learning tends to become.

The Category Test (Reitan & Wolfson, 1993) can serve to illustrate these points. Following the examinee's response, immediate feedback informs the person in no uncertain terms whether the response is correct. The feedback is deterministic: each time a response is correct a bell rings, and each time it is wrong a buzzer sounds. These are excellent conditions for learning from experience, and most examinees benefit greatly from the feedback, performing well above chance level. Further, if normal individuals were given the chance to take the Category Test again and again within a brief period of time, many would rapidly move toward very high levels of accuracy.

Imagine, however, a situation in which feedback is often no longer an easily distinguished bell or buzzer but something that perhaps sounds a little more like a bell than a buzzer or a little more like a buzzer than a bell. Imagine further that in many instances feedback is delayed, perhaps by minutes or hours or days, and that in the interim intervening events might occur that could alter the seemingly simple association between response accuracy and feedback. For example, in some instances some distorting influence might occur which leads a response of 2 to be misrepresented as 3, with feedback given accordingly. Imagine if, in addition, the feedback is systematically skewed in some fashion; for example, if the examinee is repeatedly informed that a certain type of misconception is instead correct. Imagine further that at times, perhaps more often than not, no feedback is given at all. Obviously learning via experience would become much more difficult, and one might welcome a community of scientists mounting a concentrated effort to unlock the keys to the Category Test.

We do not think it is overstating things to say that a clinician who depended solely on experience to learn malingering detection would be faced with much the same conditions as someone trying to learn under conditions of sporadic, skewed, delayed, noisy, and all too often misleading feedback. In many, if not most, instances, the clinician does not receive feedback on the accuracy of positive or negative identifications of malingering. When feedback is obtained it is often delayed, ambiguous, and skewed or distorted. If the clinician falsely diagnoses brain dysfunction, it would be the rare event for someone who is malingering to correct the misimpression. If the clinician falsely diagnoses malingering, then a plaintiff's sincere claims of disorder have not been believed in the first place, and subsequent sincere disagreement, should the plaintiff learn of the clinician's conclusion and have a chance to dispute it, are likely to be similarly rejected. The outcome of a courtroom trial, should the case be one of the small percentage that ever get that far, does not necessarily indicate the true answer, and can be contaminated by the clinician's own input. Although a clinician who believed the claimant was sincere might be confronted at trial with a videotape that provides convincing evidence that the practitioner was fooled, it establishes little other than judgmental fallibility rather than perfection, something that all but the most foolishly arrogant already recognize.

   The attempt to identify and apply malingering indicators via experience, or perhaps to modify formally validated procedures on this same basis, encounters major obstacles. If one does not consistently know who are and are not the malingerers among those one evaluates, how can one determine the relative frequency of potential indicators across the target and nontarget groups? Even if such identifications are possible in some cases, absent a representative sample of cases, as opposed to the sample and distribution of cases the clinician happens to see in his or her setting, differential frequencies may be substantially misrepresented. An accurate appraisal of these differential frequencies is necessary to determine whether a sign is useful, just how useful it might be, how it compares with other signs, whether it should be included with other available predictors, and how it is to be combined with other predictors. As the Chapmans' original research (Chapman & Chapman, 1967, 1969) and much work thereafter has shown (Nickerson, 2004; Wedding & Faust, 1989), it can be very difficult to determine the association between variables, such as potential signs and disorder, in the course of clinical practice and observation. We are prone to forming false associations between signs and disorder and overestimating the strength of associations.

   If and when valid signs are identified, one then wishes to adjust, as needed, the manner in which they are used or the cutting scores that are applied in accord with the relative frequencies of the target and nontarget populations in the setting of utilization. A decision rule that is effective in a setting with a very high rate of malingering will probably lead to far too many false-positive identifications if applied unchanged within a setting with a much lower frequency. As we will take up in greater detail later, decision rules should be adjusted in accord with frequencies or base rates in the setting of application (Meehl & Rosen, 1955). Optimum cutting points shift depending on the frequency of conditions.

   The task that faces the clinician who tries to learn malingering detection via experience is thus as follows: The clinician needs a way to determine true status, determine the differential frequency of the target and relevant nontarget groups in the setting of interest, obtain representative samples of these groups, separate the valid and invalid signs through adequate appraisal in these groups, and then devise a proper means for combining the range of valid predictors that have been uncovered, preferably by considering such matters as their nonredundant contribution to predictive accuracy and the extent to which predictions should be regressed. To say the least, this is a formidable task. It is also one that creates a blueprint for researchers.

   Some readers have undoubtedly pondered the various parallel problems that researchers routinely encounter in studies on malingering. For example, in many studies one cannot determine the true status of group members with even near certainty (e.g., whether those in the "malingering group" are really malingering). The same conditions required for learning through clinical experience need to be met for learning through research, and to the extent that studies fall short, the pragmatic help they can provide to clinicians will be compromised. Of course, this does not justify the stance that, because such conditions are imperfectly met by one or another investigation, one can then resort to experiential learning in which one routinely compounds, to a far greater extent, the methodological shortcomings of research studies. We will address various problems that researchers face at length below, but would note here that the parallels are not complete. As is well known, researchers have a range of methods that may neutralize, attenuate, or gradually lessen impediments to learning or the enhancement of knowledge (e.g., greater opportunities to gather appropriate samples, use of control groups, implementation of various procedures to attenuate bias, opportunities to alter variables systematically, and greater luxury of trial and error learning).

2　Potential Benefits of Experience and Case Study

The preceding statements should not be confused with the view that clinical experience and impressions are of no use. Rather, it is important to recognize the strengths and limitations of such evidence. Perhaps the foremost concern with case study and related methods is one of sampling. As we will argue, sampling problems often also plague other research methods for investigating malingering, but they are especially acute with case study methods and typically render attempts at generalization on this basis alone as unwise, if not unwarranted and potentially irresponsible. Despite this critical limitation, it is also the case that clinical observation has led to brilliant insights, and it is sometimes hard to imagine how such ideas could have evolved in any other context. It seems almost pedantic to say that all forms of evidence do not serve all masters equally well. When evaluating malingering research, we need not apply criteria rigidly across a diverse set of contexts where they are not fully or at all appropriate. A related error would be assuming information that meets evaluative criteria in one context will do so across other contexts without considering the shift in epistemic standards that may be necessitated by context and intended use.

Although the distinction is somewhat artificial and the boundaries not always clear-cut, it is still helpful to distinguish what Reichenbach (1938) referred to as the context of discovery and the context of justification. To detect malingering, the clinician needs efficacious predictors. Of course, predictors that no one has ever thought of cannot be validated or applied. Surely no philosopher of science would suggest that the researcher "only identify potential predictors that are known in advance to be highly valid"; we are aware of no method for doing so and such a prescription would impossibly hinder investigation. More reasonable epistemic advice might be something like, "Test your best ideas or conjectures about potential predictors, and try to avoid potential predictors that have very little chance of success, unless you are totally impeded, or unless improbable indicators, should they pan out, are likely to be very powerful; but don't inhibit yourself too much because it's hard to anticipate nature and occasionally a seemingly outlandish idea turns out to be highly progressive." In the context of discovery, one exercises considerably greater leniency when evaluating the possible merit of ideas.

One of course prefers ideas that are more likely to be correct because it is correct answers we are seeking and because economy of research effort is extremely important (there are only so many scientific hours and dollars to be spent on any particular problem). However, it is often very difficult to make such judgments at the outset and, again, our ultimate knowledge and procedures will be no better than the ideas we have thought of and tested. In the context of discovery, one might say that the only requirement is that the idea or method or sign might work, not that it will or does work, and at least for now the scientist has few or no formal methods for deriving probabilities (although Faust and Meehl (1992) have worked on these and related metascience problems; see also Faust (2006, 2008)).

If anecdotal evidence, case studies, and naturalistic studies of "caught" malingerers are viewed mainly within the context of discovery and not verification, we will be in a better position to benefit from their value in uncovering variables or indicators that may prove discriminatory, or in providing the needed grist for the verification mill. However, when the value of evidence is mainly limited to the domain of discovery, it is helpful to recognize and acknowledge these limitations, just as it is unfair to criticize a researcher whose intent is discovery for failing to meet stringent tests of verification. Often these restrictions and cautions are not limited to anecdotal evidence and its close cousins and are mainly a matter of degree, because research on malingering using more advanced designs also suffers from varying levels of concern about representativeness or generalization. More broadly, to the extent evidence or research designs may generate information of potential value but do not permit informed determinations of generalization, they might be thought of more as an exercise in the context of discovery versus verification.

3   What Is the Nature of the Phenomenon We Are Trying to Measure?

3.1   Fundamental Components

It is not an academic exercise to ask, "What is the true nature of the thing we are addressing when we refer to malingering?" This is not a question of definition, which is not too difficult (and, by itself, often resolves no important theoretical issue). Instead it is a question of proper conceptualization of external (real-world) correlates, and in particular whether we are referring to an artificial conglomeration of attributes and behaviors as opposed to something with taxonicity or internal coherence. How are we to think about the clinician's task if we do not have a reasonably clear idea about just what it is we are trying to identify? For example, the inferences and conclusions we should draw from data can differ greatly depending on whether malingering or falsification represents a continuum, or if falsification in one domain bears a high versus negligible correlation with falsification in other domains. If plaintiff Jones falsifies an early history of alcohol abuse, how much does this tell us about the likelihood he is also misrepresenting a fall down the stairs? If falsification is minimally related across domains, it tells us little; but if it is highly interrelated, then knowing that Jones underestimates his drinking by 50% could practically tell us that he fell down three steps, not the six he reported.[1]

In conceptualizing what malingering might be, at least two components seem to be required. One dimension involves misrepresentation of one's own health status (defined broadly) and the other intentionality. Whether the clinician wants to become involved in examining both dimensions, and whether the practitioner thinks that intention can be evaluated, are separate considerations from whether intentionality is needed in a conceptualization of malingering, which it almost surely is. For example, we would not want to identify a severely depressed patient who misperceives her functioning in an overly negative way or a patient with a parietal tumor who claims his right hand is not his own as malingerers.

One might also wish to parse intentionality into the subcomponents of purposeful or knowing action and the aim or end that is sought. Pretending to be disordered to obtain an undeserved damages award would not seem to equate with pretending to be sleeping so that one's 6-year-old child does not find out it was her parent and not the tooth fairy who left the dollar under the pillow. Or to illustrate the point with perhaps a more compelling or pertinent example, there is a difference between someone fabricating a disorder in an effort to avoid responsibility for a vicious crime and a crime victim feigning death to save his life. One of the difficulties here is unpacking the ontologic and moral issues. On the one hand, there might well be differences between individuals who fake illness for altruistic or at least neutral reasons as opposed to those who do so for self-gain and despite knowing their actions may harm an innocent individual. On the other hand, such distinctions between honorable and dishonorable reasons for malingering may lack objective grounding and can become rather arbitrary or almost purely subjective. For example, the same hockey player who fakes injury to draw a major penalty may be a villain in the visiting arena and a hero in the home arena, and it does not make much sense to say the justifications for the player's actions change during the flight from Montreal to Toronto. One might contrast this circumstance to a situation in which an individual plans and carries out a brutal murder for monetary gain, is caught, and then feigns insanity.

Some social scientists think that these types of value judgments are arbitrary or irrelevant, but assuredly the courts do not share their views. The normative purpose, or at least regulative ideal, of the legal system is to resolve disputes fairly, and this indeed often involves moral judgments and questions of culpability. Individuals' intended goals or reasons for doing something and the legal/moral correctness of their acts frequently decide the outcome of cases. An abused woman who feigns unconsciousness to avoid physical injury is likely to be judged quite differently than an abusing husband who fakes incapacitation so as to lure his spouse into a trap and harm her, even though both are intentionally faking disorder.

---

[1] To reduce the use of the cumbersome "he or she" or "his or her," we will alternate back and forth or vary references when we refer to gender, including the use of "they."

These value issues involve such considerations as whether there would seem to be a morally just versus immoral reason to malinger; whether the malingerer's motives are altruistic, neutral, or self-interested; and whether the act of deception comes at cost to others or victimizes them. Hence, in considering the dimensions of malingering, one might need to ask not only whether the act of providing false information is intended, but also what the individual intends to accomplish and is willing to do given an awareness of the possible consequences for others. Such judgments may reflect societal perceptions for the most part and in some instances are arguably relativistic. Nevertheless, there may well be an intrinsic, qualitatively different dimension one taps beyond falsification and intention when one looks for differences between individuals who will and will not violate major societal norms or engage in deceit for moral versus immoral reasons. Whatever the case, we will mainly limit our focus here to the first two dimensions of intent and misrepresentation.

In legal cases, there is another element that must be considered, although it does not belong on a list of candidate dimensions for malingering. In tort law, a determination of culpability, and the assignment of damages, often depend not only on the presence and extent of harm but also on cause. Smith may be terribly damaged, but if it is not the car accident but the 20-year addictive history that accounts for lowered scores on neuropsychological testing, then the driver who carelessly hit him may owe nothing for neurocognitive maladies.

A plaintiff claiming brain damage may not need to fake or exaggerate disorder at all to mislead the clinician into adopting a conclusion favorable to her case. For example, the plaintiff can simply try to mislead the clinician about cause by hiding or covering up alternative factors that explain her difficulties. Plaintiffs may also overstate prior capabilities to create a false impression about loss of functioning. Whether these alternative forms of deceit represent a separate qualitative dimension or just another phenotypic variation of a genotype is difficult to say, but there is no question that clinicians desire methods for identifying these sorts of deception as well. In fact, attempts to lead clinicians down the wrong causal path may be one of the most common forms of falsification in legal settings and deserves researchers' careful attention.

A definition of malingering that requires intention does not speak to the position or belief that malingering is or can be unconscious. From a legal standpoint, it is not clear how much of a difference there is between fooling oneself and attempting to fool others. Whether a person should be compensated for a supposed act of self-deception is a matter for the courts and juries to decide, and whether mental health professionals should enter into this particular fray is not easily answered and arguably a matter of not only theoretical viewpoint but also pragmatic feasibility (i.e., is the distinction possible to make, especially at an adequate level of scientific certainty?).

Here, what is being sought or accomplished and its justification may be central, such as whether it is the attention of others, reduction in responsibility, or absence from a stressful job; and if changes in circumstances are connected to the event in question and merit financial compensation. For example, if one somehow is using an accident as a means for assuming the sick role to solicit care and attention from a generally neglectful spouse and to avoid tedious household responsibilities, it is questionable whether someone else should shoulder the cost. In contrast, suppose a person who must drive some distance to work is struck head on by a drunk driver and suffers a severe and prolonged psychological disorder. The injured party stops driving and becomes more dependent on others for emotional support, including a spouse who views emotional maladies as intolerable weaknesses or laughable excuses for skirting personal responsibilities. The injured individual, who is perfectionist and rigid by nature, also has great difficulty accepting personal or psychological faults. In contrast, physical explanations may be far more acceptable to her and her spouse, and she voices physical complaints and perhaps develops beliefs about physical disorders the accident has caused that help accommodate shortcomings and limitations in her functioning that are causally related to the accident. To highlight the differences in these situations another way, one can ask the old Ronald Reagan question: "Are you better off today than you were yesterday?" It is hard to conceptualize an outcome that allows one to avoid what one wants to avoid and pursue what one wants to pursue and be compensated for it (i.e., in which the array of secondary gains far outweigh losses) as comparable to a circumstance in which more enjoyable or favored activities are discontinued and the less pleasant but essential ones now absorb almost all of the individual's energies.

3.2 Malingering Is a Hypothetical Construct

Malingering is a hypothetical construct. It is not a physical entity or an event in the way we normally think of such things (although it of course has an ultimate physical substrate), both of which are classes of variables that potentially can be reduced to a set of observations. The recognition of malingering (or its various forms) as a hypothetical construct carries with it certain methodological implications. First, it is not directly observable but rather must be inferred from a set of observations. To move from observations to constructs requires what philosophers of science refer to as surplus meaning (e.g., assumptions, theoretical postulates, and methods for relating or interconnecting these components). There is understandable concern about not getting too far removed from the observational base or speculating without constraint whatever the scientific data. However, the notion that to go beyond what is directly observable and infuse meaning is a methodological crime (as, say, Skinner seemed to think) is to disregard the commonplace in science. Scientific fields make broad use of hypothetical constructs (some of which later are discovered to be physically identifiable entities), and there is no direct way to go from a set of observations to theoretical constructs, a fatally flawed notion in the early positivist movement and subsequently acknowledged as a mistake. As is sometimes said, one spends the first half of a basic logic class studying deduction and the second half violating it when studying induction, but in science moving from fact to postulate and theory requires the latter.

The nature of the entities we are studying should shape our methodology. For one, if we are dealing with hypothetical constructs, operational definitions are vacuous. The obsession of some psychologists with this defunct and untenable notion of operational definitions—the remnant of a bad idea, almost universally rejected from the outset in the field in which it was proposed—is puzzling. Do we believe we could properly define such things as "quality of life" or "the best interests of the child" operationally? Do we believe if we develop five ways of measuring temperature that we are measuring five different things? Do we believe if a test contains one question, "Are you introverted?" that introversion is what the Introversion Test measures? What conceptual or scientific issue is resolved if we proceed in such a manner? Essentially none. It is worthwhile to seek clarity of language or definition, but this is different from believing that some important conceptual matter is or can be addressed by developing an operational definition. Unfortunately, a close cousin to overvaluation of operational definitions is proposing diagnostic criteria for identifying malingering that are premature given deficiencies in the scientific knowledge base, particularly when they are applied in legal settings (despite what may be clear warnings and cautions by the creators). (For further discussion of diagnostic criteria for malingering, see the final section on caveats.)

The nature of the entities we are studying and the resultant impact on appropriate methodology for *developing* assessment methods needs to be unpacked from the methods that will be most effective in *interpreting* the results these assessment tools generate. It is easy to conflate the two issues. Even if surplus meaning, inference, and theoretical considerations are essential in the development of assessment methods, this does not mean they will also be essential or important when interpreting the outcome these methods generate. For example, theoretical developments and scientific advances might result in an index that provides a simple cutoff point or probability statement. It is not coincidental or contradictory that Meehl, who together with Cronbach (Cronbach & Meehl, 1955; see Faust, 2004) radically impacted the development of assessment methods by emphasizing construct validity (versus blind or pure empiricism), also did more than anyone else to lay out the advantages of statistical or actuarial decision methods (Meehl, 1954/1996; see also Waller, Yonce, Grove, Faust, & Lenzenweger, 2006). One may maximize effectiveness by emphasizing conceptualization and theory in the development of methods, but relying on statistically based methods to interpret results or predict outcomes. Such interpretive or predictive methods need not be processed through the lens of a theory or mediated by theoretical assumptions about mind or behavior. It is commonly just assumed that if methods rest on theory or conceptualization that interpretation of the resultant output should also be based on theory or understanding, but there is no logical reason to form this link. We may need advanced theories of biochemistry to develop markers of certain diseases, but the result may be a test that yields an output that can be interpreted using a simple cutoff score. There is a related common but unwarranted assumption that the nature of the thing being appraised and the form or characteristics of measurement should resemble one another, a matter to be taken up momentarily.

3.3 Distinguishing Between the Nature of Entities and Effective Measurement Strategies

Anyone with at least a dash of scientific realism would likely agree that measurement should ultimately be dictated by external reality; that is, measurement is intended not to construct but rather to reflect what is out there. Therefore, what malingering is and is not will have major impact on the success of different approaches for measuring it. To illustrate the interrelationship between ontology (the nature of things) and measurement, if malingering truly represents multiple dimensions that are largely independent of one another as opposed to a few core characteristics with strong associations, the features of effective assessment tools will likely differ.

It would seem that we encounter an obvious circularity at this point. Measuring devices should fit the nature of malingering, but we do not yet know the nature of malingering and need effective measurement to obtain this knowledge. Hence, it would appear that we need to know more than we know if we are to learn what we need to learn. Under such conditions, how can we proceed? Here again, pseudo-positivism or operationalism will only confound the problem and not get us very far.

Within science (and within the course of human development for that matter) we often encounter this dilemma of needing to know more than we know in order to progress, and yet we frequently find some way around it. In science, this often involves some fairly crude groping around in the dark and a good deal of trial and error (Faust, 1984). We can usually determine whether we are getting somewhere by examining classic criteria for scientific ideas, such as the power to predict and, most importantly and globally, the orderliness of the data revealed (Faust & Meehl, 1992; Meehl, 1991). A phrase like "orderliness of the data" might seem vague and circular, but it has clear conceptual implications among philosophers of science and is probably the most generally accepted criterion for evaluating theories. Circularity, although indeed present, is not that problematical so long as it is partial and not complete (see Meehl, 1991, 1992). The relation between knowing the nature of malingering and measurement is dialectical—the development, ongoing evaluation, and modification of malingering detection devices ought to be based on what we come to know about malingering (our ontological knowledge), whereas our capacity to learn about malingering depends on the state of our measurement tools (our methodological or epistemological competence). Hence, knowing or attempting to know what malingering is and measuring or attempting to measure it necessarily proceed in mutual interdependence.

Although the nature of entities impacts powerfully on the success of different measurement approaches, there is hardly a one-to-one relationship between them. There is often a tendency to conflate ontological and epistemological issues. Ontological claims involve beliefs about the nature of the world or what exists, and epistemological claims involve beliefs about methods for knowing or for learning about the nature of the world. To what extent ontological claims dictate epistemological positions in an idealized system or whether the two should parallel each other is not a simple matter. However, in the practical world the two need not be isomorphic and can differ or diverge considerably without creating problems, despite what intuition or common sense might seem to suggest. For example, although the entities we intend to measure may be highly complex, this does not necessarily mean useful measurement of them must take complex forms. A few or even a single distinguishing feature may serve to identify a complex entity or condition with considerable accuracy, and at least in the short-term there may be little basis for using complex or multidimensional measurement, especially if the latter is premature and thus relatively ineffective.

Similarly, gross simplification may come very close to reflecting nature accurately (e.g., conceptualizing planetary motion as an ellipse). One might think that because the human brain and mind are complex, prediction must necessarily take into account that complexity and a myriad of data. It may be true that maximizing predictive accuracy ultimately requires that many or all of these complexities are captured, but at present the attempt to do so may create more noise than true variance and make things worse than more simplified approaches. For example, either using past behavior to predict future behavior, or merely predicting that someone will do what most people do, may work far better at times than detailed psychological assessment that attempts to appraise many characteristics or provide deep insights into a person's psyche. Assumptions about features of the human psyche (e.g., that it is complex and involves multidimensional interfaces)—or, more on point, about malingering—do not necessarily dictate measurement that mirrors these features in order to achieve the highest level of accuracy under current conditions.

Given the state of our knowledge at present and perhaps for years to come, there are times that simplifying approaches work as well or better than more complex attempts at measurement, because the latter have limitations that may introduce more error than true variance or dilute stronger predictors by including weaker ones (see the later section on attempting to integrate all of the data and the noncumulative nature of validity). Additionally, deeper understanding of phenomena or causal mechanisms may lead to the development of more sophisticated measurement approaches with decreased or minimal surface resemblance to the things being measured. Who ever imagined that the color of fluid in a tube could tell us whether someone is pregnant, that enzymes might reflect cardiac compromise, or that faint radio signals might provide critical information about the origins of the universe? Thus, the prospect that statistical frequencies might facilitate conclusions about malingering, sometimes much more so than other forms of measurement or understanding, should not lead to premature or reflexive rejection, nor to consternation. Given the importance of what we are trying to accomplish, we should embrace advances whether or not they fit our preconceptions or cognitive aesthetics.

A related questionable or fallacious belief about isomorphism, which was briefly addressed above, is that prediction must be generated by theory or understanding. One can believe that construct validity and conceptual understanding are often indispensable in test development, yet also maintain that highly effective use or application of measures can be largely atheoretical. There is a *massive* literature on prediction in psychology and related fields showing that statistically based decision procedures almost always equal or exceed clinical judgment and thus are superior overall (see Dawes, Faust, & Meehl, 1989; Faust, Ahern, & Bridges, 2011). If theory or understanding is so essential in reaching conclusions or generating predictions in psychology, then many of these studies should have come out otherwise, especially considering that, once developed, the application of statistical prediction is formulaic and not theory driven or derived. (This is distinct from arguing that good judgment in the selection, use, and application of such methods is not needed, which it is.)

Psychologists who do not distinguish between approaches for developing and appraising tests versus methods for applying them or generating conclusions will often raise ideological arguments that fail to intersect with pragmatic outcomes. For example, in many circumstances heterogeneous measures are better predictors than narrow or more homogeneous measures. A neuropsychological measure that requires multiple functions simultaneously will tend to be much more sensitive to brain damage than one that taps narrower or select capacities, although one may learn little about the specific areas of difficulty involved. If the immediate clinical task is to determine whether brain damage (or dementia, malingering, or some other particular condition or outcome) is present or likely, the selection of the heterogeneous scale might be far and away the most effective and hence the best choice. However, if one adheres doggedly to the notion that prediction should start with understanding or theory, a scale with a diverse mix of items might seem like something to be avoided assiduously. Another but converse form of ontologic-epistemologic isomorphism is to take an atheoretical approach not only to prediction but also to test development and appraisal (as hard-core behaviorists or empiricists once commonly did), something that some strong medicine from Cronbach and Meehl (1955) went a long way toward alleviating. In summary, unwarranted assumptions about ontological and epistemological isomorphism can unnecessarily restrict and impede our efforts to improve measurement.

As follows, the nature of malingering and its relation to needed or preferable measurement approaches may deviate from common belief or expectation. For example, if malingering is a category, one might falsely assume it cannot be identified by scales measuring the amount or extent of some quality (i.e., quantitative standing). However, imagine we were trying to determine whether animals fit the category of zebra. Suppose someone developed a formula that calculated the proportion of white (W) to black (B) and the proportion of white plus black to color of any type (C). If W:B and W + B:C both fall within certain ranges, the animal is to be classified as a zebra. In fact, depending on the animals being considered, such a quantitative index might work rather well, perhaps exceeding 90% accuracy. In turn, despite being based on these relatively isolated, phenotypic characteristics, the ability to identify or classify zebras with a high level of accuracy might then provide a foundation for productive research on the animal and the development of a considerable knowledge base. With a new animal, if one merely calculated the formula, the result might indicate that this knowledge base likely applied (because one was dealing with zebra), in turn permitting one to tap into a good deal of useful information or predictive power. It might take years for scientists to come up with a clearly superior method of identification, but meanwhile this quantitative procedure, an exercise in approximation or oversimplification, could serve a very useful purpose. We might finally note that effective classification rules, or even knowing whether they are effective, often follows the reverse order, that is, they come after the development of fairly extensive knowledge rather than precede it.

Key Questions About the Nature of Malingering

At present, the key ontological question seems to be whether, at the one extreme, the phenotypic variations of malingering reflect a few basic, interrelated dimensions that have substantial consistency across situations, persons, and falsified conditions or whether, at the other extreme, we are dealing with multiple independent dimensions and loose conglomerations of behaviors that change depending on the person, situation, and condition being feigned. (If we had to place our bet, it would be that malingering consists of multiple distinct categories that may or may not co-occur, and that in addition there are also dimensions of exaggeration or falsification that are not categorical.) Moving from ontology to epistemology, a key measurement issue is the development of methods that, to the extent possible, retain discriminatory power across persons, situations, and variations of falsification, and under conditions in which examinees learn their underlying design. Finally, we consider the key interface between conceptual and measurement issues to be the clinical discriminations of greatest relevance, which are those that the practitioner is required to make but cannot easily accomplish.

If malingering does have at least two basic components, falsification and intentionality, with more than minimal independence from one another, it follows that we need to capture both to identify malingering properly. Furthermore, as we will take up in detail later, any satisfactory method for identifying malingering must account for not only the presence and degree of malingering but also the presence and degree of true injury. To state the obvious, malingering and true injury are not mutually exclusive but can co-exist and are partly independent of one another. Sometimes it is one *versus* the other, but other times it is one *and* the other. If we lose sight of the fundamental difference between opposing and conjoint presentations, research in the area will never approach its true potential and will fail to address pressing legal, social, and moral needs. We contend that one of the largest and most important gaps in our scientific knowledge about malingering involves such combined presentations.

In the original version of this work (Faust & Ackley, 1998), we emphasized the value of taxometric analysis (Meehl, 1995, 1999, 2001, 2004, 2006 [specifically Part IV]; Waller & Meehl, 1998). These methods, which require modest to relatively large samples, serve to clarify the latent structure of variables and are well suited for work on malingering. In addition, even absent definitive or near-definitive methods for identifying group membership (e.g., those malingering versus those not malingering), the methods provide means for identifying optimal cutting scores and estimating base rates. There has been a gradual increase in the use of taxometric methods in malingering research, and it has sometimes supported the existence of distinct categories (as opposed to underlying dimensions) (e.g., Strong, Glassmire, Frederick, & Greene, 2006; Strong, Greene, & Schinka, 2000) and sometimes has not (e.g., Walters et al., 2008; Walters, Berry, Rogers, Payne, & Granacher, 2009). We think expanded work with such methods promises to add much to our knowledge about categorical versus dimensional status and classification.

Finally, attempts to examine the categorical status of malingering should avoid artificial constraints on its manifestations. Many malingering studies present subjects with only a few measures or options. Although there is nothing wrong with this per se or when conducting certain types of studies, restrictive response options can create fatal problems when one is trying to capture the nature or structure of malingering. In the clinical situation, a potential malingerer has a wide range of options and is almost never forced to fake on a predetermined, narrow range of tests. Rather, the malingerer can fabricate history and symptoms and may well be selective in faking test performances. If the researcher severely restrains the range of options for malingering and forces the individual to fake on a specific or narrow set of measures, a very distorted picture of malingering may emerge. It would be analogous to attempting to determine the underlying characteristics of the dolphin's sensory system by solely measuring whether sound can be detected at a certain level, or to examining the works of Robert Frost by only counting the average number of words in a sentence. None of this should be confused with an argument for considering or integrating all possible evidence in assessing malingering (which is often counterproductive advice; see Faust, 1989, and subsequent material in this volume). Rather, an attempt to determine underlying structure should provide the opportunity for the phenomenon to manifest itself as it is and should not artificially, and severely, constrain its expression.

4 Clinical Needs and Research Agenda

Recognition of the noteworthy gains made in malingering detection should not obscure the considerable challenges that remain. Rather than accept our current tools as good enough and think that, even if there are gaps in research, clinical experience and judgment can almost invariably overcome remaining limitations, we can ask what the most pressing research needs might be. It seems sensible to argue that, all else being equal, the cases that remain most difficult to detect or classify set the main clinical agenda, which in turn sets the main research agenda. Although essentially going hand in hand, such research should also focus on improving or augmenting the best measures and methods, or extending their reach, and not on creating more methods or approaches with validity, but that offer no particular advantages over currently available methods. As straightforward as this seems, a large volume of research may not be directed precisely toward the most pressing clinical needs.

Given the scientific advances that have occurred, a certain percentage of cases are now easily identifiable and can be classified with considerable accuracy. However, in many other instances the clinician's task remains challenging, and more advanced research knowledge and appraisal methods are needed. These remaining difficulties may be obscured or underappreciated exactly because much research does *not* examine these more challenging (but common) presentations and thereby can yield a misleading picture of overall efficacy. Whittling down the percentage of remaining ambiguous or difficult cases will almost surely become progressively more trying and will likely require protracted effort. As we gain more success, those individuals who remain difficult to identify are generally harder and harder cases, and thus the scientific challenges increase accordingly.

There is obviously minimal need for additional research on the types of cases we can identify almost flawlessly. We seemingly should concentrate instead on those cases that frequently exceed our current capacities or knowledge. In general terms, the latter sorts of cases are often those for which there are reasonable grounds to suspect malingering, and one must make the distinction between those who are suspected of malingering and are malingering versus those suspected of malingering who are not malingering. This differentiation is usually far more difficult than distinguishing between cases in which there is almost no reason to suspect malingering versus those in which the evidence for malingering is overwhelming. Yet research is often conducted with these easily identified groups. How informative is it to study very distinctive groups we know how to identify with near certainty in order to learn how to identify those we do not know how to identify (precisely because they lack the distinguishing features of the easily identified groups)? Viewing the main research agenda as cutting into the percentage of difficult to identify or ambiguous cases, we will first discuss the groups of greatest interest, then cover factors that may contribute to false-negative and false-positive errors, next compare clinical needs to common research strategies, and finally present a series of research suggestions.

4.1   Framing the Problem

There is almost nothing more important for advancing malingering research than to identify representative samples of cases. Were this possible, it would greatly facilitate efforts to uncover distinguishing features, such as the characteristics that separate individuals for whom there is a good basis to suspect malingering and who are and are not malingering, and go a long way toward deriving accurate base rate information. In pursing such aims, it helps to clarify the groups of interest or the individuals who make up the relevant population or subgroups. Figure 2 reflects an attempt to frame this population.

The focus of Fig. 2 is on litigants. We realize that falsification or malingering is not of concern solely in legal cases, but given the main aim of the current text and volume, Fig. 2 is directed toward forensic groups. Further, the characteristics of

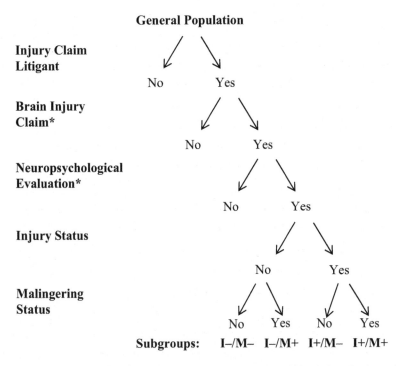

General Population

Injury Claim Litigant

No   Yes

Brain Injury Claim*

No   Yes

Neuropsychological Evaluation*

No   Yes

Injury Status

No   Yes

Malingering Status

No   Yes   No   Yes

Subgroups: I–/M–   I–/M+   I+/M–   I+/M+

Fig. 2 Identifying relevant subpopulations in forensic neuropsychological evaluations. (*The order of these steps can be reversed and outcome of the neuropsychological evaluation can influence whether a brain injury is claimed.)

litigants are of greatest relevance for neuropsychological evaluations and research within that arena. The materials that follow are arguably narrower than the overall legal domain because most of our commentary is related to the civil arena, and there are probably important differences or distinctions between civil and criminal cases. For example, in a civil case a major issue may be the occurrence of brain injury and its future consequences. In a criminal case the main concern may be retrospective, such as whether months earlier during a murderous act the defendant's pre-existing brain injury impeded the capacity to form criminal intent or control behavior at the time of the crime.

As illustrated in Fig. 2, some litigants will claim brain injury or dysfunction, and some of this group will be seen for neuropsychological evaluation. In some cases brain injury is suspected but does not become an element of the case until a neuropsychological evaluation generates an abnormal result. The evaluation may have been initiated in the context of treatment or arranged by an attorney. For the moment, the main point is that, for the neuropsychologist, the overall group of interest is not litigants as a whole or all litigants claiming brain injury but litigants who may or will claim brain injury and who are being evaluated by a neuropsychologist. The importance of all this is that information about the other groups, such as all litigants, will usually be of little or no relevance to research on malingering detection within neuropsychology in the legal or civil context. Whether the base rate for malingering is, say, 5% or 25% for litigants overall, it matters not a whit because that is not the group that neuropsychologists evaluate in the legal context, and it is the base rate of malingering in the latter group that matters. Similarly, when one thinks about a representative sample or the subcategory from which to try to derive such a sample, the relevant group is not litigants overall, but it is those litigants that neuropsychologists evaluate.

As critical as it is to distinguish between the subgroups in Fig. 2 and their relevance to clinical and research efforts, this figure is an exercise in oversimplification. For example, for the entry, *Neuropsychological Evaluation*, there may well be differences among individuals examined by a treating neuropsychologist, the plaintiff's neuropsychologist, the defense's neuropsychologist, or across two or all of these contexts. Possible distrust of the "opposing" neuropsychologist could lead to systematic differences in evaluation results on average. Furthermore, no attempt has been made to distinguish between such factors as the magnitude or type of injury, the potential presence of co-occurring or independent conditions, the amount of money at stake (e.g., $50,000 versus $10,000,000), or litigants' sociodemographic characteristics. There may also be regional differences and differences based on the type of claim or forum (civil, criminal, family court, adult versus juvenile). The mixture of individuals can also change over time. For example, the frequency of cases in which mild brain injury is being claimed can change over the years for a number of reasons (e.g., perhaps a few lawyers have highly visible success with such cases, certain kinds of cases repeatedly bring poor results, or awareness of mild head injury increases due to media and medical attention to war-related or sports-related concussions).

Given these complexities, when a specific base rate is cited for malingering one wonders about its basis, merits, and value, in particular because *general* base rates are often of little help and, rather, one seeks base rates that are narrower and more specifically applicable. To illustrate the point, the base rate for Alzheimer's disease for the overall population is much less helpful than the base rates for a group whose age is comparable to that of the patient, especially if one is dealing with a 7-year-old versus a 70-year-old patient. (The importance of using base rates that are as narrow as possible is discussed later.) The more one considers these sorts of complexities and their implications, the more apparent it becomes that we have often just brushed the surface of clinical and scientific issues crucial to this area.

The flow chart depicted in Fig. 2 is obviously limited to coarse groupings, although in many circumstances even such broad separations may be missed, potentially dooming attempts to get at greater specifics almost before one gets started. The rows labeled *Injury Status* and *Malingering Status* do not reflect a temporal or diagnostic sequence or hierarchy. Rather, they are separated in the flow chart to distinguish them conceptually. We wish to avoid what sometimes seems to be a "versus" bias in this area, or the tendency to treat these categories as if they were exclusive of one another more often or to a greater degree than is warranted. Combining injury status and malingering status, we end up with four subgroups (i.e., not injured and not malingering; not injured and malingering; injured and not

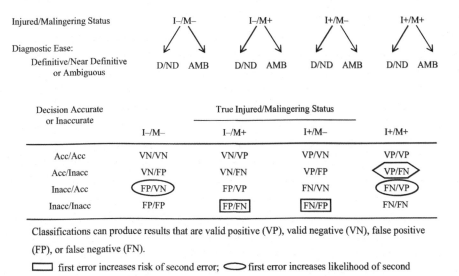

| Injured/Malingering Status | I–/M– | I–/M+ | I+/M– | I+/M+ |

Diagnostic Ease:
Definitive/Near Definitive
or Ambiguous

D/ND   AMB   D/ND   AMB   D/ND   AMB   D/ND   AMB

Decision Accurate or Inaccurate	True Injured/Malingering Status			
	I–/M–	I–/M+	I+/M–	I+/M+
Acc/Acc	VN/VN	VN/VP	VP/VN	VP/VP
Acc/Inacc	VN/FP	VN/FN	VP/FP	VP/FN
Inacc/Acc	FP/VN	FP/VP	FN/VN	FN/VP
Inacc/Inacc	FP/FP	FP/FN	FN/FP	FN/FN

Classifications can produce results that are valid positive (VP), valid negative (VN), false positive (FP), or false negative (FN).

▭ first error increases risk of second error; ⬭ first error increases likelihood of second correct identification; ⬯ the first correct decision increases risk of the second error

Fig. 3 Types of cases, diagnostic difficulty, and classification of decision accuracy

malingering; and injured and malingering). We have represented all four subgroups using dichotomous divisions to simplify this illustration, but we know that the real situation is more complex and nuanced.

Figure 3 takes the four subcategories arrived at in Fig. 2 and divides the cases within each into those that can be identified definitively or nearly so (D/ND) and those that are more ambiguous and difficult to identify (AMB). As we have emphasized, the nexus of both clinical and research needs is the AMB case. Furthermore, we think that far more research should be directed toward the falsifying *and* injured group (I+/M+). We will return to the four subcategories in Fig. 3 when we compare the match between areas of greatest clinical need and commonly applied research designs. For now, we will examine factors that contribute to case difficulty and that help to pinpoint areas of research need.

4.2 Sources of Inaccuracy

Figure 4 illustrates some of the important distinctions clinicians commonly must consider when appraising the accuracy of information. Information about the examinee's condition can range along a continuum that extends (at least hypothetically) from completely accurate to completely inaccurate. Inaccuracies can arise from various factors, including not only misrepresentations stemming from the individual but also from such sources as measurement error. It would immediately seem clear that we are never, or almost never, at either end point of the continuum, but rather some place in between; that is, we operate with some balance of accurate and inaccurate information.

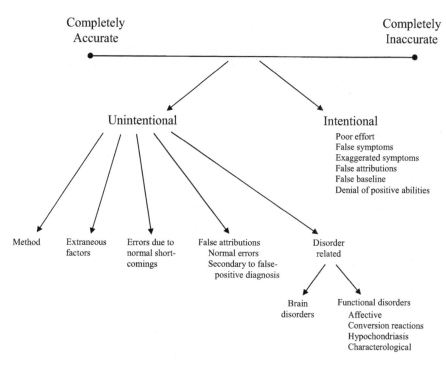

Fig. 4 Sources of inaccuracy in assessment data

Inaccuracy can be intentional or unintentional (although we realize that some individuals would place intentionality on a continuum as well). In this context we are not using the term *unintentional* to refer exclusively to a mental state, but rather in a more general sense to encompass various sources of inaccuracy in neuropsychological data, none of which anyone sets out to find or create. For example, inaccurate information can stem from problems with methodology (e.g., measurement error, misadministration of tests). Inaccuracy can also result from the operation of extraneous factors that contaminate the data or lead to results that misrepresent the patient's more typical or characteristic state, such as poor sleep the night before the evaluation, a flare-up in medication side effects, or a transient poor mood that impedes the examinee's efforts.

Other unintentional forms of inaccuracy originate from the examinee. Some are disorder related. For example, brain damage may impair insight, as when a grievously injured patient reports minimal difficulties in everyday functioning. Functional or personality factors and disorders, including normal human shortcomings, can also lead to misreporting. After all, who has perfect insight into their own strengths, weaknesses, and personal characteristics? Some individuals characteristically or stylistically under- or overperceive their capacities. Persons with affective disorders may underestimate their behavioral and cognitive capabilities and overperceive their functional difficulties. Individuals with conversion or somaticizing disorders may believe they are brain impaired when they are not, or that they are more incapable or impaired than they are, and they may misperceive normal behavior as indicative of disorder, skewing their self-reports. False-positive diagnoses may lead examinees to mistakenly believe that they are brain-damaged and to greatly overestimate the frequency of neuropsychological difficulties, and false-negative diagnoses may lead to the opposing types of errors in self-perception and self-reporting. Some individuals reconstruct an overly positive image of preaccident functioning and may misperceive their present normal shortcomings as pathologic or as representing a change in status (Mittenberg, DiGiulio, Perrin, & Bass, 1992). Consequently, they may describe a long list of "symptoms" secondary to their injury.

People can easily form false attributions about the causes of their problems (if these judgments were always so easy, there would be little need to consult highly trained specialists to determine etiology). The patient with dementia who has started down the path of progressive decline may suddenly come to the attention of service providers after a mild head injury causes a temporary diminution in cognitive functioning, with subsequent problems blamed entirely on the car accident. The patient who shows persisting symptoms may attribute them to medication side effects rather than the head trauma, the patient who cannot concentrate at work may blame the problem on exposure to toxins rather than a sleep disorder, and so on. Clinicians usually ask patients to discuss possible precipitating factors and may give great weight to their self-reports, sometimes above all other information. (It would be fascinating to study the frequency with which patients draw correct conclusions about the causes of their conditions when there is no incentive to mislead but powerful incentives for accuracy.) Considering the many ways examinees can inadvertently mislead themselves and others, it would be outrageous to assume that any type of misrepresentation provides strong evidence of malingering; this is exactly why we cannot overlook the element of intentionality.

Intentional inaccuracy or misrepresentation can take various forms. For example, the examinee may make a poor effort on testing, may make up symptoms, may overstate symptoms, may purposely cover up or mislead about causality, may present a false baseline, or may fail to acknowledge strengths, positive abilities, or positive areas of functioning.

The pragmatic task facing the clinician (and the researcher) would not be nearly as hard if the array of available information tended to show powerful interrelationships. Were this the case, then if one could identify a few pieces of information or variables that could be classified accurately, one would usually be able to predict or determine the category within which much of the remaining data would fall. For example, were malingering on the Dr. Soothsayer Inventory strongly predictive of malingering on all other tests, clinical life would be relatively easy. However, it is because interrelations are so imperfect that we are usually surprised when virtually everything in an assessment lines up in just the same direction and the case becomes as trivially obvious as it is atypical.

We do not intend to review factors that often produce low relations among various measures of accuracy in self-report and test behavior (e.g., measurement error, differences in the validities of variables measured, selectivity in what is falsified), but the point remains that it is present. Consequently, being able to classify results accurately on one particular test or variable frequently does not allow one to predict the classification (or determine the underlying explanation) of other data points. Even though we do not necessarily obtain high associations across measures and areas, we would still like to know the strength of relations between variables. At least then we would be able to intelligently address the question, "Knowing the correct classification on variable(s) A (B, C, and D), what can I predict about classification on other variables or groups of variables?" Furthermore, knowledge of such interrelations can help direct our attention toward combinations of variables that show the broadest predictive power, that is, variables that show the strongest loadings on the dimensions or qualities that represent malingering. Knowledge of interrelationships is also critical in combining variables to draw overall conclusions about cooperation or lack of cooperation with assessment procedures, something that is often neglected or evaluated inaccurately, potentially resulting in costly or devastating judgment errors.

Some clinicians, having obtained powerful evidence for suboptimal performance on one measure, may select the default option and conclude that most or all other results are placed in doubt or that they reflect minimal capacities. On the obverse side of the coin, having obtained unremarkable results on one or a few "malingering" tests (which are often structurally similar to other tests in a battery on which an individual may have performed unremarkably), another clinician might conclude that good effort has been exerted across the battery. Structurally, such a broad generalization about good effort seems as or more risky than one relating to inadequate effort because a commonly advocated approach is to set very high cutoff levels for identifying malingering. In either case, the clinician is moving from one or a few samples of good or poor effort on the examinee's part to generalizations about level of effort or cooperation across the entire battery, a practice that is often further compounded by the decided tendency for accuracy rates obtained in initial studies to diminish considerably in applied settings (see the later discussion of the extreme group problem). Given these considerations, it seems apparent that a far better understanding of the interrelations between results on measures of malingering and effort, as well as the various measures of neuropsychological functioning included in batteries, would be very helpful in applied clinical and forensic work. The frequency and degree of independence among these various dimensions are among the more fundamental reasons the injured and malingering (I+/M+) group is of such importance and a major research priority.

More generally, the clinician must consider such sources of inaccuracy as methodological ones (e.g., measurement error), transient factors, individual and personality factors, forms of pathology that can lead to misrepresentation, inadvertent false attributions, and the various forms of intentional falsification that might occur. Some of these possibilities are likely to influence performance or reporting in select domains, and others are likely to have a wider impact. For example, an inadvertent causal misattribution is unlikely to have much influence on test performance, whereas an intentional effort to portray memory deficit is likely to affect the patient's self-report, the history she provides, and test performance. Furthermore, the clinician would like to know, should he obtain definite or strong evidence about level of effort or accuracy on one or a few variables, the extent to which generalizations can be made about the genuineness of the dysfunctions reported or observed in other areas and about information pertaining to cause.

In the planning and design of malingering research, it is helpful to maintain a broad appreciation of these sorts of complex determinations the practitioner faces. The practitioner wants to be able to separate an individual with a conversion reaction who has experienced a mild head injury and who genuinely believes she has memory difficulty but does not, from one who has experienced a mild head injury and who had memory problems but has subsequently recovered and is now faking deficit. Or the clinician may be trying to differentiate between an individual with moderate head injury who has serious memory difficulties, has organically based motivational problems, and, because of affective disorder, tends to overperceive his level of difficulty, as opposed to one who in fact has mild memory difficulties but is claiming and portraying moderate-to-severe memory problems. It is understandable that many malingering studies have examined simple distinctions as a way of getting started. However, it will be very important to extend the scope of this research to these more complex differentiations that are commonly required in clinical and forensic practice.

4.3   Factors That Contribute to Case Difficulty and Ambiguity

Various factors can contribute to case ambiguity and make the appraisal of deception challenging, a number of which appear in Table 1. We certainly do not contend that this is an exhaustive or definitive list, and we recognize that some items overlap or are not mutually exclusive. However, it seems apparent that research aimed at reducing the frequency of ambiguous cases should focus on these sorts of variables. For the most part, we have placed items under respective categories based on whether they relate most importantly to the examiner, the examinee, or high-priority research needs. Some entries could arguably be placed in a different category or in multiple categories. For example, "Conditions less well studied" is listed as an examinee factor but is certainly also a general research need. For organizational purposes, we have limited entries in the category, "Additional Factors/High-Priority Research Needs," to items that, as the designation suggests, are both especially critical research topics and are minimally covered or not covered at all under other general categories.

For some of the entries in Table 1, the most likely resultant error is a false-positive identification, for some it is a false-negative identification, and for other entries both types of errors tend to be produced. For example, if an individual has a worse than typically expected outcome, the likelihood of a false-positive identification of malingering increases; if an individual is an especially skilled fabricator, the likelihood of a false-negative error increases; and mixed or complex presentations

Table 1 Factors contributing to case difficulty; sources of false-positive and false-negative errors

Examiner factors	
Data gathering and selection of procedures	Interpretive approaches
• Weak or poor tests and methods • Combining weak methods with stronger methods • Inadequate coverage • Timing/placement of measures • Over-testing or overly lengthy sessions • Poor match in conditions or sociodemographic features • Testing while examinee in fluctuating states • Testing during flare-ups of co-occurring features, associated conditions, or extraneous conditions (e.g., headaches, medication side effects, seizures, sleep disorder, pain, mood disorder) • Inadequate data collection (e.g., information about prior functioning)	• Confirmatory bias, premature closure • Illusory correlation, inadequate covariation analysis • Overconfidence • Inappropriate disjunctive or conjunctive strategies • Trying to integrate all data, adding weaker predictors to stronger predictors, viewing validity as cumulative, insufficient attention to incremental validity • Focusing on complex pattern analysis • Selection of or overreliance on weaker interpretive methods, subjective judgment; underreliance on validated/statistical decision procedures • Countervailing validated interpretive procedures too readily • Failure to consider or properly apply base rates • Unwarranted generalization • Misappraisal of injury severity • Disregard of other factors compromising effort • Bias/advocacy
Examinee factors	
• Skill at falsifying • Preparation/"coaching"/incentives • Overlap • Fluctuations or changes in condition • Flare-ups of co-occurring features, associated conditions, or extraneous factors • Attentional lapses/poor concentration • Complexity (e.g., number of co-occurring conditions, number of factors producing inaccuracy, injured and malingering) • Either worse or better than expected outcome • Other factors compromising effort (e.g., mood disorder, rapid fatigability, low frustration tolerance)	• Conditions less well studied (e.g., electrical injury, rare toxin) • Absence of hard evidence • Intra-individual variation • Cultural diversity • Other factors compromising accuracy of self-report (e.g., memory dysfunction, lack of insight, severe mood disorder) • Subtlety of presentation/relevant differentials • Indirect causal chain between event and outcome
Additional factors/high-priority research needs	
• Insufficient knowledge about mixed presentations • Extreme group problem (e.g., qualitative and quantitative shifts) • Lack of representative samples	• Misleading base rates (e.g., under- or overestimates, improper subgroups) • Transparency of methods; extending half-life • Data combination methods, knowledge of differentiating value, incremental validity

may lead to an increase in both false-negative and false-positive errors. The entries are not in any presumed order of relative importance, and, as noted, we certainly do not suppose the list is exhaustive or that we have identified all important sources of error.

Others could add to the list and might consider alternative factors greater priorities, although we do believe we have identified various important sources of error. Whatever one's exact choices or preferences, if the central aim is to reduce the percentage of ambiguous cases, identifying sources of error is not an exercise in self-flagellation but serves as a helpful starting point to highlight practice and research priorities.

Examiner factors are further subdivided into data gathering and interpretive functions. Most of the factors involve avoidable error or underutilization of available scientific knowledge that can help reduce error and optimize accuracy. Some of these factors simply involve procedural missteps, such as excessive testing that may result in lowered motivation and effort among genuinely injured individuals that is then mistaken for malingering. It is probably apparent that the list could be expanded (e.g., scoring error, misadministration of measures). However, our intent is not to cover everything that might go wrong in an evaluation but rather to highlight certain factors that may require increased attention or that perhaps are not intuitively obvious.

Particularly for those entries bearing on interpretation, much of the needed fundamental scientific knowledge base does not await development but already exists, and the issue is far more one of recognition and utilization. Thus, one might say that the problem is commonly one of education, training, and application rather than insufficient scientific foundations. Fortunately, this body of knowledge in decision making is readily available and there for the using. Unfortunately, not only is this information regularly underutilized, but intuition and common beliefs within the field frequently run contrary to more effective practices, thus diminishing decision accuracy compared to what is achievable. For example, as will be discussed later, the notions that it is usually best to combine large amounts of information, that such information can be synthesized as a whole, and that validity is cumulative lead to practices that often compromise accuracy. We will emphasize problematic interpretive practices that may be less self-explanatory or less generally recognized. Additionally, some of the caveats appearing at the end of the volume further address the application of decision research in reducing examiner error. Detailed discussion of this body of literature and its positive applications is available in various sources (e.g., Arkes, 1981; Faust, 2007; Faust et al., 2011; Faust, Arkes, & Gaudet, in press; Wedding & Faust, 1989; see also Waller et al., 2006, Chapter 8 which reproduces Meehl and Rosen's [1955] classic article on the use of base rates and Chapter 9 which provides guiding examples for application of this material).

4.4   Examiner Factors: Data Gathering and Selection of Procedures

In Table 1, two interrelated procedures appear first under the heading, "Data gathering and selection of procedures." Obviously, selecting weaker procedures (e.g., the Rey 15 Item Test) over stronger procedures is almost a sure way to reduce accuracy. The limited survey data on preferred approaches for appraising deception are not reassuring and suggest that frequency of use sometimes bears little relation to level of validity (Sharland & Gfeller, 2007; Slick, Tan, Strauss, & Hultsch, 2004). At other times, stronger methods might also be used, and it might be assumed that weaker components cannot really hurt and may contribute a modicum of useful information. Perhaps these weaker procedures are used because they require minimal time or cover a domain that other measures do not address, or they may be applied as a screening tool to determine whether more detailed assessment is needed.

A good deal will be said later about beliefs that underlie data collection and integration, and particularly the common but counterproductive assumption that validity is cumulative (i.e., the more information the better). Despite the sometimes broad acceptance of this viewpoint and its general appeal, it is contradicted by fundamental psychometric principles and a great deal of research evidence. Were such an assumption about more necessarily being better true, then, for example, if one had 10 measures that each accounted for 15% of the variance, one could potentially account for 150% of the variance. Furthermore, given the error rates associated with psychological tests, when multiple measures are used it is almost inevitable that some of the results will represent error and thus will flat-out contradict other results that are accurate. Studies indicate that in many circumstances, a relatively small set of predictors (perhaps 3–5), if properly selected, will often approach or reach a ceiling in predictive accuracy. At that point, adding further predictors, especially weaker ones, will not improve the situation. The weaker the measure, the more likely and more often it will conflict with stronger measures, and hence to the extent it influences decision making, it will tend to degrade overall accuracy, sometimes substantially. In an area like malingering detection, in which there are often multiple measures with respectable psychometric properties, failing to add one measure to a group of effective measures usually has minimal negative impact, whereas combining weak predictors with more effective ones may have a sizeable negative impact. As a rule of thumb, when a range of sound procedures or tests are available, errors of omission are less costly than errors of inclusion.

Using brief (and often weaker) methods as screening devices is often, simply put, poor practice. Each individual who is not malingering but fails the screening becomes a potential false-positive error, and each individual who is malingering but passes the screening is almost sure to become a false-negative error. In the latter instance, results on the screen are used to decide whether further evaluation is needed, and hence a false-negative error is unlikely to be reversed. The ultimate result is that a weak screening device that frequently misclassifies individuals is an almost sure bet to increase error as opposed to starting with a stronger method.

The sensible desire to save time by starting with a brief screen is often overwhelmingly offset because better alternatives may not require much greater time and, more so, because of the stakes involved.

Suppose, for example, one uses a poor screening measure (e.g., the Rey 15 Item Test), which in some circumstances has at least a 50% false-negative rate, and further suppose one is evaluating mental competence in a murder case. Here, at least half of the malingerers will not be detected and, therefore, will not be subject to further formal appraisal of falsification. Additionally, the measure may also be prone to false-positive errors with the most severely impaired individuals. Even if further testing is conducted, the result from this poor test may still have a sizeable impact on clinical decisions. Earlier information in an assessment, all else being equal, may have a greater impact on judgment than later information by shaping or channeling the manner in which subsequent information is interpreted. A related practice is to only administer a test of effort if one suspects malingering based on clinical impression. Given what is known about the limits of clinical judgment for appraising malingering in comparison to other methods, such a screening strategy is as bad or worse than using weak measures. When operating in areas in which the evaluative task often poses challenges and the stakes are high, one should start with the strongest measure if at all feasible, especially if the outcome is used to decide whether additional evaluation is needed. In the context of what may be a lengthy neuropsychological evaluation spaced over a number of days, if one is going to screen for malingering, it is almost always far more effective to use a method that might require an extra 10 or 20 min but is considerably more accurate than a briefer measure.

To illustrate the consequences of a poor screening device, assume one measure has a 50% false-negative rate and a 15% false-positive rate (test A: 50/15) and another measure a 20% false-negative rate and a 15% false-positive rate (test B: 20/15). Assume that test A requires 10 min and test B 20 min. Now suppose that 100 individuals are evaluated and that 50 of them are malingering. For purposes of simplification (and because it will not change the basic point being illustrated here), we will focus on the 50 malingerers. If we use test A first, 50% of the malingerers (or 25 individuals) will be missed and will not be subjected to further testing. The remaining 25 are then administered test B. Given test B's 20% false-negative rate, 5 are misclassified, which, when added to the 25 prior errors results in 30 total misses or a 60% error rate, which of course is worse than chance.[2]

In contrast, if one uses only test B, of the 50 malingerers, 10 are missed, resulting in a 20% error rate. (In reality, given typical psychometric relationships, although it might seem as if administering test A next would reduce error further by avoiding some of the false-negative errors of test B, it is likely to worsen the false-positive

[2] For purposes of illustration, we have treated Method A and Method B as completely nonredundant. Usually the situation is more complex and there is some degree of interdependence, which makes it even worse to use a weak screening measure or add weak measures to stronger measures. For example, a weaker method may "correct" some of the errors a stronger method makes, but it will "spoil" the correct conclusions of the stronger method a greater number of times.

rate an equal or greater amount and hence should be avoided. For a further explanation, see the subsequent materials on data integration.) One might then ask what the
cost is in time or money of using the latter method and reducing the error rate by a
factor of three. If we start with test A, the 50 malingerers require 500 min in total,
and the 25 individuals who go on to be administered test B require another 500 min,
for a grand total of 1000 min. If, instead, all 50 are given test B only, the result is
1000 total minutes, or exactly an equal time expenditure to achieve a vastly superior
result. If the circumstances justified adding test A or another such measure of comparable length, and if the 40 individuals with positive results on test B were also
administered the second test, one would be adding a total of 400 min, or less than 7
hours across 50 total individuals. By adding an average of 8 min per individual, one
goes from 30 errors to far fewer errors. (If the analysis is expanded to include all
those with positive and negative results on the initial screening, and one assumes all
those with positive results are administered the second test, the additional time
expenditure remains rather modest.) If the screening measure showed a propensity
toward false-positive errors, the change in accuracy might not be as dramatic, yet
the percentage of damaging errors might still be reduced considerably. In the context of neuropsychological evaluations that might require about 10 h per individual,
how would the expert explain the effort to save a few minutes on average at the cost
of a twofold or threefold increase in the probability of error? Thus, as a general
guide, if at all feasible, one should start with the best measure (and only add further
measures if they increase overall accuracy or help cut down on the most costly form
of error).

The third factor listed, inadequate coverage, refers to overlap in content areas
between standard neuropsychological measures on which performance has been
weak or poor and malingering measures. For example, suppose the clinician uses
two malingering measures that both involve visual memory tasks. Suppose, however, the examinee has performed extremely well on standard tests of visual memory functioning. What are the chances of insufficient effort in this area? The range
of options that are now available for malingering appraisal often permits the selection of one or more measures in areas in which performance is weak or poor. It is in
those areas that concerns most naturally arise about the adequacy of effort and distinguishing genuine impairment from insufficient effort. Overlap in content area is
a relatively easy subject to research and worth pursuing. For example, one could
examine the likelihood of detection if one does or does not cover domains in which
performance on standard tests was poor, or one might conduct simulation studies to
examine relations between attempts to feign in discrete areas and performance on
malingering tests in associated and nonassociated content domains. Over time, we
may be able to develop formal procedures with solid scientific foundations to select
malingering tests based on the examinee's performance on standard tests across
content domains. Although many evaluators likely use their clinical judgment to
make such selections, there are powerful reasons to believe that formal procedures
with firm scientific backing will be more effective overall (see Faust, 1993; Faust &
Ahern, 2011).

The next factor listed in Table 1, the timing and placement of measures, refers to the tendency of some evaluators to administer effort tests very early or late in the assessment sequence. Some examinees require a period of time to overcome initial anxiety or discomfort and may underperform on early measures. Should the use of measures designed solely to assess effort be avoided, initial tests may still be checked for performances that fall short of expectations for the condition in question. In such cases, the combination of distress and true injury may yield results that fall within ranges deemed suggestive of inadequate effort.

Some examiners place effort tests at the end of batteries. Individuals with any of an array of neurological and psychiatric disorders that decrease endurance or persistence may reach a point at which performance is severely compromised. Neuropsychologists may continue testing beyond the point at which performance is compromised, perhaps because the examinee does not disclose fatigue or lacks sufficient awareness of its impact, or perhaps due to the practitioner's inflexibility or worse. When combined with such factors as over-testing or overly lengthy sessions, the result may be false-positive outcomes. For example, we have been involved in multiple legal cases in which an examiner continued testing for 8 h or more on a single day and administered effort measures last. Again, because performance below expectation on standard measures may also be emphasized as a potential indicator of malingering, markedly diminished performance due to exhaustion or emotional flooding toward the end of a long day can create an additional, and sizeable risk of false-positive error. We would recommend that all examiners at least record the order of test administration. Better yet, they can record starting and stopping times for each test and any breaks during testing sessions to allow timing and placement to be examined in clinical and legal cases and for research purposes.

The remaining factors listed under data collection should be self-explanatory and, as will be the case for other such entries in Table 1, we will not elaborate on them in this section.

4.5 Examiner Factors: Interpretive Approaches

Most of the factors relating to interpretation are almost pure applications of decision-making research. A core aim of this long-standing, highly active research area is to foster greater decision accuracy and hence enhance human welfare. One avenue for achieving this end is to identify factors that impede judgmental accuracy, which sometimes assails sacred idols, but ultimately serves a constructive purpose. Increased understanding of judgmental strengths and limits helps direct the design of methods for overcoming problems and augmenting success rates. Given the considerable pragmatic help the decision literature can provide in enhancing accuracy, it is a valuable addition to the tools we can bring to clinical and forensic settings and seemingly ought to be embraced rather than resisted as is sometimes the case.

Two core impediments to greater judgmental accuracy include cognitive biases and insufficient adherence to normative judgment practices (e.g., the proper utilization of base rates). When decision researchers address biases, they may not be so much interested in emotional factors that impede clear judgment but rather in errors of "cold" cognition, that is, misjudgments rooted in mental processes that need not be fueled or activated by the distorting effects of emotion. (This is not to overlook the compounding effects that human emotions or needs may have on reasoning or analysis.) Various problematic judgment practices seem to occur even when individuals are highly motivated to arrive at the right answer, do not seem to have an axe to grind, and are not influenced by strong emotions. To provide an example, in as simple a situation as one in which individuals try to uncover the underlying principle in an ascending string of numbers (e.g., 2–4–6–8), they usually try to confirm rather than disconfirm their hypotheses. As is well understood, under certain circumstances, this is an inefficient and potentially misleading strategy. For example, one might hypothesize that the underlying principle for "2–4–6–8" is an increase in the numbers by 2 and guess "10–12–14" for the next several numbers; but if the correct underlying concept is ascending numbers by *any* amount, the false hypothesis will be confirmed each time. If one instead tried to *disconfirm* the hypothesis by guessing 9, the resultant feedback would be more informative. There seems to be a fairly broad range of "cold" cognitive biases. When they are uncovered and found to have a detrimental influence on judgmental accuracy, researchers seek ways to intervene and foster better decision-making approaches.

Confirmatory Bias and Premature Closure

Confirmatory bias refers to a series of problematic judgment practices with a basic common feature—the tendency to maintain beliefs despite what should be convincing counterevidence. Aspects of confirmatory bias include "favoritism" toward one's initial hypotheses, inconsistent standards for evidence depending on whether it tends to support or refute one's beliefs, and premature closure, or the tendency to form initial hypotheses quickly and on the basis of limited information. Greenwald, Pratkanis, Leippe, and Baumgardner (1986), and Nickerson (1998) also describe research showing selectivity in recalling information that appears to support one's assumptions. Confirmatory bias may exert considerable impact, and has been the subject of many studies with both laypersons and professionals, including those in mental health fields (for an overview of this literature, see Nickerson, 1998). Such biases typically occur without our realizing they are operating.

Premature closure refers to the tendency to draw initial conclusions too rapidly (Galanter & Patel, 2005; Nickerson, 1998). In an earlier study, Yager (1977) found that psychiatrists frequently formed diagnostic impressions of patients within the first *2 or 3 min* of contact, and sometimes in as little as *30 s*. Insufficient delay before forming beliefs increases the likelihood of starting off on the wrong track, and thus can worsen problems created by other types of confirmatory bias. Resistance to reconsideration of initial impressions is obviously the opposite of what is needed when correction is required. The term premature closure connotes that once initial impressions are formed, they tend to remain unaltered—one becomes shut off to new evidence.

Confirmatory bias can also alter data gathering. Information that supports one's hypothesis is often more likely to be collected than negative information, even if the latter is as or more plentiful and available (Arkes, 1981; Nickerson, 1998). If confirmatory bias can lead to the underweighting of negative evidence, this problem will become more acute if nonsupportive data are less likely to be gathered in the first place. In addition to biases in gathering information that supports hypotheses, forensic examiners may influence the behaviors of examinees such that they tend to elicit, or in some sense artificially create, the very evidence they seek. (Terms to describe such occurrences include *channeling effects* and the more familiar *self-fulfilling prophecy.*)

Obviously, in malingering assessment all of these types of biases could operate. For example, forensic evaluators may select instruments with greater or lesser tendencies to produce false-negative or false-positive errors, may form powerful initial impressions that shape subsequent data collection and interpretation, or may act toward litigants in ways that elicit behaviors or reactions that seem to confirm their impressions. Additionally, when referring attorneys make initial contact with experts, there is a risk that the information that is conveyed or the manner in which it is presented can skew impressions and get the process started off on the wrong track.

There has been very little formal research on the potential operation of confirmatory bias in the assessment of malingering, or on possible corrective methods within this context. More general research on corrective methods (e.g., Arkes, 1981; Faust, 2007) suggests that confirmation bias is attenuated by actively considering alternative hypotheses or explicitly recognizing negative evidence that might be present or available. The most powerful protection, however, is the use of systematic procedures for data collection and interpretation that are less likely to be affected by premature clinical impressions or initial hypotheses. For example, by relying mainly on structured procedures for gathering information, one should be less susceptible to the potential impact of confirmation bias that could lead to insufficient probing of certain background factors, such as the range of skills needed to perform certain work requirements. Similarly, if one uses a well-validated, formal decision procedure when interpreting a test result, biases are less likely to impact the process. Additionally, one should be especially cautious (as opposed to freewheeling) before countervailing the outcome of a well-supported decision procedure, actively consider the evidence that supports the procedure's outcome, and limit rejections to usual or compelling circumstances.

Illusory Correlation and Failure to Analyze Covariation

As coined by the Chapmans (1967), *illusory correlation* refers to the tendency to form false conclusions about the associations between variables or to overperceive the strength of association. For example, an examiner may believe that certain nervous mannerisms are suggestive of attempts at deceit, whereas they may be no more common among malingerers than nonmalingerers and reflect ordinary reactions to situations in which so much is at stake. Considerable research points to the regularity with which many mental health professionals form false associations (e.g., see Herman, 2005; Nickerson, 2004), and the aforementioned survey research on malingering detection strategies, which suggests heavy reliance on weaker methods, strongly implies that illusory correlations are frequent in this area, a rather disconcerting thought.

The formation of illusory correlations often starts with insufficient covariation analysis. To properly determine whether a relationship is present between variables (e.g., between a clinical finding and malingering), one must determine whether the finding occurs more frequently when malingering is present than when it is absent. Without the full set of facts—the presence and absence of the indicator when the condition *is* present and when it is *not* present—the determination cannot be made. Appraising these four conditions, or analyzing covariation, is one of various ways to evaluate whether variables are truly associated.

Individuals often have considerable difficulty evaluating covariation and thus commonly draw false conclusions about relationships (e.g., Arkes & Harkness, 1980; Nickerson, 2004). In particular, they tend to overweigh or attend mainly to the frequency with which the sign of interest co-occurs with the condition of interest. Table 2 provides a simple illustration. Here the diagnostic sign is the presence of what the clinician considers a "red flag" for malingering, such as long response latencies. Cell A refers to the "sign present and condition present" situation, which often draws the most attention (red flag present and malingering present). Laypersons or clinicians often also consider one of the other cells, such as cell B ("sign absent and condition present"), but they frequently fail to consider *all* of the cells (A through D). However, short of considering all four cells, or lacking trustworthy information about all the cells, one cannot determine whether a true relation exists between the sign and the condition.

Of course, in the area of malingering detection, although one can often determine whether the sign or indicator is present, one frequently lacks a clear way to determine if malingering is present (especially with ambiguous cases). This is one of the main reasons experience may have such limited benefits in this domain. How can one appraise whether one is forming accurate judgments or illusory correlations if one cannot consistently determine whether the condition of interest is present or

Table 2 The four cells of a covariation table

Condition (Malingering)	Sign ("Red Flag")	
	Present	Absent
Present	A Sign present Condition present	B Sign absent Condition present
Absent	C Sign present Condition absent	D Sign absent Condition absent

absent? To make matters worse, how could one even begin to determine whether one is observing a representative sample of cases and thus has the data needed to perform a proper analysis?

Many interesting possibilities have been raised as potential malingering indicators, which generally coincide with common sense or assumptions. Numerous sources provide lists of potential "red flags," some with good support, some with a little support, and some that have never been formally tested and yet may be described as if they had been well established or validated. There is considerable potential benefit to generating such candidate variables because some of them may be of substantial value, but it is very concerning that they often seem to be applied before any formal scientific appraisal has occurred and, furthermore, that they may be used in lieu of indicators or methods that have been validated. Even if a number of these proposed indicators have validity, this does not mean they will lead to greater accuracy when combined with other valid and perhaps more powerful variables, and they could lead to a decline in accuracy by diluting the impact of superior variables. (These unintended consequences are likely to occur regularly because validity is not cumulative.) Virtually all of these potential variables, even those that would appear to be purely qualitative, can be quantified (e.g., $1 = present; 0 = absent$) and subjected to formal study. In the meantime, it would be very helpful if those proposing such lists were very clear on the degree and type of support for items and their demonstrated efficacy (if any) so that professionals considering them could make properly informed decisions.

Overconfidence

Overconfidence is among the most pernicious judgment problems and may well be prevalent in malingering evaluations (e.g., Faust, Hart, & Guilmette, 1988), partly because we lack proper corrective feedback and partly because conditions in research studies often produce inflated accuracy rates (see discussion of the extreme group problem below). Absent clear feedback or, in many cases, receiving no feedback about accuracy in identifying malingering, how does one adjust one's level of confidence appropriately?

The extensive literature on confidence and accuracy often distinguishes between two dimensions. The first dimension is the relation between confidence and accuracy. For example, research may indicate that as clinicians become more confident they also become more accurate. The second dimension is referred to as *calibration* and addresses the degree of concordance or divergence between confidence and accuracy. For example, someone who is 50% confident may be accurate about 50% of the time, when 70% confident may be correct about 70% of the time, and so on. When level of confidence and level of accuracy are appropriately aligned, the individual is said to be well calibrated. In contrast, there may be a marked disparity between level of confidence and accuracy. Someone else may be correct only about 10% of the time when 50% confident, and correct only about 30% of the time when 80% confident. Note that this individual does show some association between confidence and accuracy—when he is more confident, he is more accurate—but his calibration is poor given the considerable gap between level of confidence and accuracy. Because these two dimensions—the association between confidence and accuracy, and calibration—are partly independent, they often need to be considered separately in research on the topic.

Studies of mental health (and other) professionals commonly demonstrate a weak or even negligible association between confidence and accuracy, and improper calibration as well, with overconfidence being the typical finding (e.g., Elkovitch, Viljoen, Scalora, & Ullman, 2008; Faust et al., 1988; Faust, Hart, Guilmette, & Arkes, 1988; Garb & Schramke, 1996; Guilbault, Bryant, Brockway, & Posavac, 2004; Herman, 2005; Nickerson, 2004; Sieck & Arkes, 2005; Wedding, 1983). Nickerson (2004) describes overconfidence as an "occupational hazard" in fields that do not provide clear feedback about the accuracy of judgments, which of course applies to malingering detection. (For a classic discussion about how overconfidence develops among mental health professionals, as relevant today as it was when written, see Hyman, 1977; for a discussion of factors that converge to foster overconfidence, see Faust & Ahern, 2011.)

Overconfidence is associated with numerous adverse influences on decision makers. For example, clinicians who are overconfident tend to reach conclusions too soon, or before gathering adequate information, and may not subsequently revise conclusions even when new evidence should be convincing. Overconfident professionals underuse helpful decision aids and corrective methods. Suppose a clinician who, in truth, is 60% accurate believes he is 90% accurate. Consequently, he may reject a decision procedure that research shows achieves 80% accuracy, even though it could cut his error rate in half (from 40% to 20%). Similarly, decision makers who are overconfident countervail validated decision procedures too often. For example, a scientifically sound decision procedure which classifies a test result as indicating good effort may be rejected too readily by a professional who is overly sure about her clinical judgment (see further below).

Overconfidence can lead to other problematic practices, such as insufficient care when gathering data. The examiner might administer and score psychological tests without sufficient rigor and hence be error prone. Overconfident decision makers frequently show reduced openness to new developments in the profession, make inadequate effort to seek or appraise negative evidence, and tend to make overly extreme predictions. Despite ambiguous data, an overly confident clinician may, for example, feel certain that a criminal offender with a history of violence is not malingering and recommend early release without reservation.

Overconfidence is closely tied to confirmatory bias. Evaluating hypotheses by focusing on supportive evidence is likely to inflate confidence. Suppose about equal amounts of evidence argue for and against a diagnostic hypothesis that Mr. Smith is brain injured, and further assume, given this mix of evidence, that the hypothesis will be correct about 50% of the time. A clinician who primarily seeks out and focuses on the supportive evidence is likely to feel more than 50% confidence that the condition is present and may develop a level of conviction that far exceeds the likelihood of being correct. As with confirmatory bias, one mental habit that may attenuate overconfidence is deliberate consideration of reasons one's conclusions might be wrong (Arkes, 1981). If our clinician reached a tentative conclusion that Mr. Smith was brain injured and not malingering, he might re-examine the patient's file for evidence that suggests this conclusion is incorrect, or he might actively consider or attempt to generate viable reasons an alternative conclusion might hold. The patient, for example, may have exhibited a month or so of seemingly normal functioning after the accident. Confirmatory strategies may dominate routine clinical appraisal, and hence a deliberate strategy of *considering the opposite* can make contrary information more salient and thereby lead to appropriate readjustments of confidence levels.

Inappropriate Disjunctive or Conjunctive Strategies

Some examiners identify malingering if any measure is outside acceptable limits, and some do not identify malingering if any measure is within acceptable limits. Both of these disjunctive strategies are usually unwarranted and not based on any formal body of literature for combining results across the tests. Perhaps most concerning, both approaches are almost sure to produce an increasing frequency of error the greater the number of malingering measures that are used because the errors across the tests will compound one another. For example, if test A has a 10% chance of a false-positive error, test B a 15% chance, and test C a 15% chance, then the likelihood of at least one scoring falling above the respective cutoff is obviously greater than 15% (although by how much depends on the level of redundancy across the measures, which may never have been formally analyzed). Consequently, although it can be said the approach is psychometrically unsound, just how badly it performs is often unknown. The same problem applies to the opposing disjunctive strategy and the resultant false-negative error rate, in which case the likelihood of at least one score falling below the malingering cutoff is some joint product of the various tests. Not knowing how well a method operates precludes proper calibration of confidence in conclusions and makes one wonder how the expert can provide an informed opinion about such a vital matter when operating from an informational vacuum.

One sometimes sees the suggestion that one set high cutoffs for each malingering test, and, should the outcome on any such test exceed the specified cutoff, judge overall effort and perhaps all of the standard test results as questionable. Those prescribing such strategies sometimes assume they will reduce both false-positive and false-negative errors, which is highly improbable. Cut scores can be set to maximize overall accuracy, but in the great majority of cases reducing one form of error (i.e., false-positive or false-negative error) will come at the cost of increasing the opposing type of error. To illustrate this concept with an extreme, if one were to identify no one as malingering no matter the test outcome, it would reduce the false-positive rate to 0%, but of course the false-negative error rate would increase. Decision policies try to identify the most acceptable balance between false-positive and false-negative errors given a cost-benefit analysis, but they are not premised on the untenable belief that one can simultaneously minimize *both* false-positive and false-negative errors. It is true that improved decision-making procedures can reduce the amount of error overall and thereby, in comparison to weaker decision methods, might lower both the false-positive and false-negative error rates. For example, a decision procedure that yields an overall accuracy rate of 60% may result in 20% false-positive and 20% false-negative errors, whereas one that produces an 80% accuracy rate may result in 10% false-positive and 10% false-negative errors. However, for either of these policies respectively, if one adjusts the cutoff score to reduce one form of error it will almost inevitably increase the opposing form of error.

The kind of disjunctive strategy that has been suggested, which raises cutting scores per test to try to reduce the overall false-positive error rate, will partly realize that outcome compared to a disjunctive strategy that sets lower cutting points per test. However, lacking knowledge of the redundancy among tests, it still might lead to an unacceptably high level of false-positive errors. For example, if an examiner uses five different measures with limited redundancy and sets the cutoff at a 90% probability across tests, the conjoint probability of a false-positive finding could still be considerably greater than 10%, such as 25% or more. Additionally, in no small part, the risk of false-positive error will merely be a product of the number of tests used, an arbitrary or inconsistent basis for determining such matters. More so, such a disjunctive strategy is almost sure to be psychometrically nonoptimal, does not produce a known accuracy rate if the tests that are used have not been studied in combination, and may deviate from optimal cutting points by a considerable margin. The likelihood that such a disjunctive approach will optimize accuracy in any given situation, instead of using alternative methods to combine the information optimally, may not be zero but it is not far from it.

Certain conjunctive strategies can be even worse than disjunctive approaches. Some evaluators require that results across all relevant tests or dimensions be above a certain level before they will identify malingering, and some that all be below a certain level before they will rule out malingering. Depending where these levels are set, the rate of either false-positive error or false-negative error can easily reach appalling levels, levels that are worse than chance and may even approach 100%.

Data Combination

Deterministic versus probabilistic framework. There are compelling grounds to argue that the most fundamental error in approaches to psychological assessment and malingering detection, and in strategies that are commonly used for combining or integrating data, can be summarized as follows: Despite the recognition among many psychologists that they are operating in a probabilistic decision domain, the processes they follow in collecting and interpreting information often rest, nevertheless, on an implicit deterministic framework. Much trouble can be traced to this source and it usually results in advice for combining information that undermines much of the advantages our hard won scientific advances have achieved. It is a little like a parole officer who knows one should look carefully into an individual's criminal history, which may include numerous serious crimes committed over decades and which scientific study shows has strong predictive value; yet being overly influenced, perhaps without full self-recognition, by the offender's facial expressions that seemingly convey deep sincerity about repenting.

Until our science is perfected, we seek the ideal but live with the real. In an idealized world of forensic evaluation, there would be a deterministic relationship between the information we gather and the outcome or condition we wish to identify. By *deterministic* we mean a perfect association between data and outcome, with no error or separation between the two. For example, the result of a malingering test would provide a definitive indicator of true status; that is, there would be a perfect association between the test result and malingering. For the moment we are addressing *methodology*, that is, the status of our methods for knowing or assessing matters (i.e., how accurate a procedure is for identifying some entity or predicting some outcome) and not the status of the physical world (e.g., whether event A is the sole cause of event B). Stated as the philosopher would, we are addressing epistemology (methods of knowing), not ontology (claims about the nature of the world).

In contrast to deterministic relationships between data and outcome, psychologists, especially within the forensic domain, deal almost exclusively with *probabilistic* relationships. By probabilistic, we mean that the data contain a certain amount of error or randomness, and hence the relation between the data and outcome is imperfect. The level of error is sometimes relatively small and sometimes large, an example of the latter being when a test result predicts an outcome at slightly above chance level. Stated in another manner, given our probabilistic situation, a very poor score on a measure of intellectual ability will not always indicate low intelligence because a different, although perhaps far less likely, explanation may apply. Perhaps the examinee made little effort on testing in a case involving death sentencing, or perhaps the psychologist felt morally compelled to underreport the result.

Although virtually any psychologist recognizes that a deterministic relationship almost never exists between obtained data and the things we are trying to identify (e.g., between a score on a malingering test and poor effort on the test taker's part), we often proceed in a way, or follow dictates, more suitable to a deterministic world. Take the following common suppositions, each one of which contains a strong deterministic element or accords more with deterministic than probabilistic thinking:

- In general, the more data the better.
- No single test or result is usually of great significance by itself; rather, most or all available information should be considered together.
- Although multiple data points and sources may seem to contain inconsistencies, skillful analysis and synthesis should permit them to be integrated into systematic and meaningful patterns.
- Pattern analysis is often fundamental for diagnostic, predictive, and explanatory purposes. For example, conditions often can be identified by their patterns on neuropsychological evaluation.
- Once one has integrated the information and deciphered underlying patterns in the data, the resultant understanding provides the foundation for determining or

predicting other important things (e.g., occupations someone may be able to handle or how well someone may perform if certain memory capacities are stressed).

The deterministic framework that underlies these and other common working assumptions might not be apparent, partly because such assumptions are so deeply embedded in our training and thinking. However, consider the notion that most or all of the data can be synthesized into a consistent whole. This assumption presumes nearly, if not entirely, error-free measurement (which basically rests on a deterministic framework). Suppose instead one assumes probabilistic relationships, and therefore fallible or weak connections, between at least some of the data points and outcome. It thereby follows that a number of these data points will probably point in the wrong direction and should not be integrated with other, correct data points. For example, assume one relies on 10 tests or indicators to evaluate malingering and that each one of them has about a 25% error rate. Consequently, 2 or 3 of the 10 indicators will be wrong on average and should not be included or "integrated" with the correct indicators.

Many commonly employed interpretive approaches do not really align with or incorporate the probabilistic circumstances we face in the vast majority of instances. Even when we seem to realize at some level that we are dealing with probabilistic data, we tend to dismiss some of the most basic methodological implications and rather approach data collection and interpretation as if the situation were deterministic. Additional examples of the disparity between the recognition of data as probabilistic and received views on the methodology of assessment in the behavioral sciences can be offered. The following two methodological guidelines follow from a probabilistic view, although they may initially seem somewhat odd or misguided:

- Excluding weaker information is often more important than gathering and considering a broad array of information.
- Various results will not only seem to be misaligned or inconsistent with each other, they truly will be contradictory. Consequently, an essential task is to decide what to exclude, rather than to uncover some explanation that synthesizes all of the information.

In summary, whatever the idealized situation or our wished-for state of future knowledge, in nearly all present circumstances in psychology and law and malingering evaluation, we work in a probabilistic world of decision making. Recognition and acceptance of our fundamental methodological situation should not be deflating; it merely acknowledges imperfection in our state of knowledge. Paradoxically and more importantly, realizing that some degree of error is unavoidable can assist us in making less error (Einhorn, 1986). This recognition frees us to adopt various approaches that will likely increase our diagnostic and predictive accuracy and thereby increase the number of situations in which we can assist the courts.

When theory-based prediction is superior. Many courtroom issues involve discrete judgments and predictions, this often being the case with the appraisal of malingering. Approaches to decision making and prediction can be separated into two basic types as a first approximation: theory-based and atheoretical. Theories can yield impressive predictive accuracy and exactitude, but to do so a series of conditions must be met. First, the theory needs to be well corroborated, with scientific laws on assumptive networks supported by a body of converging, formal evidence. Second, sufficient knowledge is needed of the factors that determine outcomes (e.g., if outcomes are mainly determined by six factors, one usually must be aware of all six). Third, there must be tools or procedures that measure standing on those factors accurately or precisely. Unless all of these requirements are satisfied, theory-based predictions will probably be compromised substantially, if not enfeebled. In psychology, we rarely meet all three requirements, and it is hard to think of circumstances in which we presently do so in malingering detection. This is not to suggest that psychologists are alone with these challenges; equal or greater difficulties are encountered across many areas of scientific endeavor.

The general absence of high-powered theories does not preclude important positive contributions in the legal domain. Even if our level of success is more modest, there will certainly be times that neuropsychological evaluation and appraisal of malingering promote meaningfully greater levels of accuracy than would be realized without expert evidence. What it does imply is that current strategies for maximizing courtroom utility and predictive accuracy might not follow commonly assumed strategies that, in reality, require more advanced scientific knowledge than we currently possess (and seek to develop over time). If we are not open to possibilities other than theory-based prediction, or prediction based on "understanding," we may overlook or reject useful alternatives because they seem incompatible with assumptions we are perhaps too ready to treat as givens. However, openness to alternatives may simply require recognition that most decision making in psychology and law occurs under probabilistic versus deterministic conditions.

In the area of malingering appraisal, what ultimately should make a difference is not whether judgment or interpretation rests on theory but how often the professional can reach correct conclusions and do so more accurately than the trier of fact.[3] Thus, although it may seem paradoxical, the utility of theories and models in developing assessment tools can be distinguished from the most efficacious ways to apply these tools or to interpret the outcomes of evaluations. For example, we can sometimes maximize the chances of an accurate conclusion by relying heavily on a base rate or a cutting score.

If we are thinking probabilistically, then our main goal is to reduce the level of uncertainty about the relation between the data and the conclusion or outcome. It should not necessarily make a difference if our current understanding of the mechanisms by which methods achieve predictive accuracy is limited. For example, one of Frederick's (2003) indices for identifying insufficient effort on the Validity Indicator Profile seems to lack an obvious rationale or explanation, but it does

---

[3] We realize that appearance will impact juries, but we do not believe this should ever override accuracy. We believe our highest priority should be to get it right, at which point we can worry about how to present our findings in an understandable manner that creates *warranted* belief in our work.

appear to be effective. Similarly, incorporating methodological or probabilistic principles into data gathering and interpretation or prediction often does not depend on adopting any specific theory about neuropsychological functioning because, in the main, one is applying knowledge about how to predict or decide. Maximizing predictive accuracy in the mental health field, given the status of theories, remains in no small part a matter of applying decision technology. We often have restricted comprehension of how or why technologies achieve desirable ends, but the absence of a sound explanation should not lead us to disregard or reject effective decision methods. We often use things in everyday life because we trust they will work (e.g., cell phones and computers), even if we do not fully understand their underlying operation. Even those most familiar with technologies sometimes lack an understanding of causal mechanisms, knowledge of which may take years to develop (as is common in medicine).

Is complex pattern analysis and integrating large amounts of information always the preferred strategy? A common corollary of the emphasis on theory and explanatory framework is the preeminent role assigned to pattern analysis, especially complex pattern analysis and data integration. We do not dispute the ontological underpinnings of such assumptions but rather the methodological program that is assumed to follow, which we think is often misaligned with the current state of knowledge and inadvertently reduces judgmental accuracy.

Many discussions of malingering assessment in texts, research articles, and test manuals describe the efficacy of methods but then advise exercising judgment in integrating all of the data or information. Reliance on clinical judgment is advised either because placing primary reliance on cumulative indices or formal procedures for combining information is viewed as error prone (as if clinical judgment were not) or because formal integrative techniques are not available for the methods the clinician has used. There is, however, a crucial distinction to be made between exercising sound professional judgment and adopting subjective judgment as the ultimate method for integrating data. For example, formalized decision rules should not be followed blindly or robotically because situations may arise that attenuate or negate their value. In one instance a child fell asleep during the administration of a memory test but the examiner nevertheless included the memory score when tallying test results. We are not aware of any intelligent advocate of formalized decision procedures who would endorse such a foolish act, but to disapprove of such mindless missteps does not provide logical support for the argument that data should almost always be integrated via subjective or impressionistic judgment. It is the difference between saying that because an animal is not an elephant it might be a bear, as opposed to concluding this means we should not brush our teeth; that is, it is the difference between a logical connection between A and B and an illogical one. More generally, we should not advocate for a decision procedure because it fits some cognitive aesthetic or commonly accepted ideology despite research evidence, but because, all else being equal, it delivers the most accurate results.

Research on complex data integrative capacities. Assumptions about the ability to perform complex data integration with high levels of proficiency conflict with a large body of research on human cognitive limitations, which can be traced back at least as far as Simon's (1956, 1957) classic work on *bounded rationality*. As the term suggests, limits in human cognitive capacity often set surprising restrictions on the ability to manage complex information and decipher relations among data correctly or optimally, especially without decision aids. Considerable research with laypersons and professionals suggests that individuals, even when functioning at or near their best, are often far less capable of managing complex information than has frequently been assumed (e.g., Armstrong, 2001; Faust, 1984; Hogarth & Karelaia, 2007; Ruscio, 2003).

The evidence for limits in the capacity to manage complex data comes from multiple converging lines of research, which will only be touched on briefly (for further details, see Faust & Ahern, 2011). One line of investigation examines clinicians' judgment accuracy when provided with various amounts of information. This work suggests that once a limited amount of valid information is provided, additional information often does little or nothing to increase judgmental accuracy, and sometimes leads to diminished accuracy (e.g., Golden, 1964; Grove, Zald, Lebow, Snitz, & Nelson, 2000; Ruscio, 2003; Sawyer, 1966; Wedding, 1983). For example, Sawyer's (1966) extensive earlier review showed that when data are combined via clinical judgment, accuracy is as good or *better* when clinicians rely on testing alone rather than a combination of testing and (unstructured) interview, a result similar to Grove et al.'s (2000) meta-analysis.

Although it might seem paradoxical that "more may be less," the explanation for such outcomes is not too obscure. Consider a situation in which you select stocks on your own and make excellent choices 30% of the time. You then seek out the advice of two stockbrokers, one who makes excellent selections 60% of the time and the other 75% of the time. Although following the second broker's advice more or less assures excellent selections in 75% of cases, you naturally would like to bolster this rate. This is the type of situation the psychologist often faces when attempting to integrate data. There may be one or more relatively strong indicators, but they do not attain a satisfactory level of accuracy when used in isolation. There are additional indicators that, although not as strong, do show valid relations with the criterion. Finally, there are usually a variety of weaker or invalid so-called indicators.

Psychologists and neuropsychologists are typically advised to integrate or combine "all of the data," but it is sometimes difficult to see how this can be done. If all indicators point in the same direction, there is no problem. However, in many cases, if for no reason other than measurement error, variables conflict. This does not necessarily reflect superficial inconsistency that deeper analysis would show to have an underlying order indicative of the examinee's true characteristics. Rather, commonly, some variables provide accurate information about the case at hand and others do not. If one variable indicates that stock A will beat stock B over the next year and another variable produces the opposite prediction, it is hard to imagine that at a deeper level the contradiction evaporates.

To return to the brokers or consultants, in some cases they will disagree. If you simply go with the broker who is right 75% of the time, you will have a 75% accuracy rate. Alternatively, you might look for exceptions, or instances in which you would defer to the other broker who, after all, is likely to be right at times when the first broker is wrong. The problem with this approach is that, at the outset at least, you have no trustworthy way of identifying exceptions, for that would usually require knowledge superior to that of the better consultant. If you had such knowledge from the start, the consultants probably would not have been needed. If, instead, you defer to your own judgment to identify exceptions, you are using a weaker predictor to override stronger predictors, a strategy almost guaranteed to fail in the long run. Therefore, at least at first, the best strategy is almost surely to defer to the superior broker in all cases. You can carefully study cases of disagreement over time to see whether certain ways of combining information from the two brokers enhances accuracy. For example, you might find that for stocks in the electronics field Broker 2 usually beats Broker 1 and, in those instances, you should generally defer to Broker 2 in cases of disagreement. Augmenting decision procedures by identifying exceptions, however, often turns out to be much more difficult than we think and frequently backfires (Faust, 1984; Grove et al., 2000; Meehl, 1986). With the present example, there is also the possibility that in almost every case, or in every case, in which the brokers disagree, the stronger broker is right and the weaker broker is wrong.

Of course, the easy solution is to go with the good data and disregard the bad data, but it is not necessarily easy to execute this intent in practice. It may not be easy to determine, especially based on subjective or clinical judgment, how robust a predictor might be or even if it is valid, as research in such areas as covariation analysis and illusory correlation suggests. Furthermore, if we accept the common dictate to integrate all of the data, it almost demands inclusion of weaker or poor data. There are surely times when obtaining additional data can contribute to predictive accuracy. The primary problem seems to rest in difficulties appraising whether predictors are valid and just how strong they may be, and then holding in mind, weighting, organizing, and integrating data proficiently (see further below).

Another line of research on the limits of data integration capacities uses mathematical procedures to construct models that reproduce clinicians' decisions. When developing models, or more specifically an individualized model for a single clinician at a time, researchers usually present case materials and ask the particular clinician to reach conclusions or make predictions, such as whether a patient is likely to act violently. Multiple cases are presented in which patient characteristics vary. Some cases, for example, describe past violent acts and others the absence of such acts. Statistical analyses examine relations between standing on the background variables or case features and the clinician's decisions. The intent is to derive a formula (i.e., a mathematical model) that reproduces the clinician's judgments as frequently as possible. To determine how well the models perform, the clinician might be asked to judge a series of new cases, the same data are entered into the model or formula, and level of agreement is examined. The analysis might or might not show a high level of agreement between the clinician and the model of that clinician. As noted, one typically builds models separately for different clinicians and examines agreement between each model and the clinician upon whom the model was based, although some work extends to group or pooled decisions.

When constructing models, researchers often start with simple approaches and build complexity as necessary. For example, one might start with simple linear composites of variables and then examine whether more complex models, such as those that account for interrelationships among data (i.e., configural relations), alter the level of agreement between model and judge. Research often shows that models can reproduce clinicians' judgments with modest to high levels of accuracy and that simple models often perform nearly as well or as well as more complex models (e.g., Armstrong, 2001; Dawes, 1979; Goldberg, 1968, 1991; Hogarth & Karelaia, 2007; Ruscio, 2003).

One has to be careful about the interpretations drawn from these studies because the models reproduce clinicians' decisions and not necessarily their reasoning processes. For example, even reproducing decisions with a high degree of regularity using simple linear models does not rule out human ability to perform any type of configural analysis. The findings do suggest, however, that decisions believed to depend on configural analysis or complex data integration can often be reproduced by simple procedures that ignore configural relationships. If decision makers routinely perform configural analyses that make unique contributions to decision accuracy, nonconfigural models should not be able to duplicate their judgments with regularity. Thus, the findings suggest that whatever configural analyses clinicians may perform often do not accomplish much above and beyond simply adding data together. On the whole, the modeling research raises serious questions about the capacity to perform complex configural analysis routinely.

Other research, much of which involves nonprofessionals, demonstrates frequent difficulties recognizing and understanding even fairly simple configural relationships, such as those involving relationships between only a few variables (see Faust, 1984; Hogarth & Karelaia, 2007; Ruscio, 2003). The results of these and other studies further suggest that the configural strategies that laypersons and clinicians implement, rather than integrating large volumes of data and deciphering complex interrelations, are often simplifying approaches that are applied to manage information overload (and accomplish this mainly by disregarding much of the information). The discrepancy between introspective analysis of decision processes and more objective measures of what really is and is not accomplished is often startling and humbling, but at the same time highly instructive.

Emphasizing incremental validity and appropriate selectivity. Maximizing decision accuracy often requires the dual tasks of identifying and emphasizing the most useful information and identifying and deemphasizing (or discarding) the less useful or useless information. Information that lacks utility or is invalid may well diminish accuracy, and thus it is commonly as or more critical to determine what information to exclude when forming conclusions as it is to determine what to include. The common advice to "integrate all available information" has a subtle erroneous component, but one with surprising potency to diminish judgmental accuracy and cause harm. These adverse consequences could be largely negated by a seemingly simple change to instead recommend that "within the bounds of ethics and feasibility, use all of the information that increases accuracy and none that does not."

This alternative principle is merely another way of describing *incremental validity* as a foremost concern. Incremental validity refers to the potential influence of adding new information to other available information. If the new information increases accuracy, it possesses incremental validity. As will be discussed in more detail later, in clinical and forensic practice, approaches for combining information on effort or malingering often seem to place insufficient (or no) emphasis on the formal analysis of incremental validity, although such practices are slowly changing (e.g., see Bain et al., 2019; Berthelson, Mulchan, Odland, Miller, & Mittenberg, 2013; Bilder, Sugar, & Hellemann, 2014; Larrabee, 2014). In addition, research on combining malingering indicators is commonly conducted under conditions in which generalization to applied settings will frequently be poor or lead to major judgment error or misleading outcomes (despite what may be researchers' stated cautions). For example, the likelihood of malingering or poor effort could be over-estimated by a large margin and contribute to settlements or verdicts that are truly unjust.

As noted, with many judgment tasks, a ceiling in accuracy is approached or reached with a limited set of the most valid and least redundant predictors, often no more than about three to five variables. There may be multiple other valid variables, but incorporating them in the interpretive process will likely yield little or no benefit (making their use inefficient) and may diminish accuracy. Additional variables are frequently redundant and hence do not contribute unique predictive information. Furthermore, if weaker predictors are combined with stronger ones, particularly via clinical judgment or impressionistic methods, the impact of the superior predictors may be attenuated or overridden and, as a result, accuracy can suffer.

When interpreting information, it is routine to emphasize validity, but the importance of redundancy may be under-recognized. All else being constant, two valid, nonredundant variables will yield greater accuracy than a hypothetical, infinite group of variables that are completely redundant with one another. Predictive accuracy is increased as one combines variables with two qualities: (1) validity and (2) unique versus overlapping (redundant) information. Suppose, for example, we are evaluating a person's physical health and can obtain two measurements. If we measure weight with an exact scale, another measure of weight using another exact scale will contribute no unique information. We would learn more by adding, say, a measure of blood pressure, because it is valid and partly independent of weight. With psychological measurement, redundancy is very rarely an all-or-none quality but the exact same principles apply—the extent of incremental validity hinges on both validity and redundancy.

One reason clinical judgment can be so challenging is that proper analysis of validity *and* redundancy, especially when multiple potential variables are involved, is very difficult to perform subjectively and cannot be expected to match formal procedures. Furthermore, as the stockbroker example was intended to illustrate and as perhaps is less well appreciated, valid variables may not only fail to produce incremental validity but may *decrease* accuracy. Thus, it is not necessarily helpful and may well be counterproductive to collect or use as much information as one can, even if all of the information is valid. Despite this psychometric truth, articles and manuals on malingering assessment continue to emphasize both extensive information gathering and utilization of clinical judgment as the ultimate means for interpreting that information.

Incremental validity should often be the primary guide for determining what information to include or exclude in decision making. In most situations, the most effective combination of variables should be identified, with no further variables added when they do not impact on accuracy positively and particularly if they decrease accuracy. This should not be mistaken as an argument for the use of tests exclusively. Considering the advantages of nonredundancy, it is entirely possible that other sources of information will contribute to incremental validity. Speaking broadly, however, we are likely to maximize overall accuracy if our determinations about seeking or including additional informational sources rest on proper knowledge of their positive or negative impact when combined with the best predictors that are already available. Of course, unless the information that is gathered is interpreted properly, it might not do us much good. What routinely follows prescriptions for gathering or utilizing most or all of the data is, as noted, the advice that its integration should ultimately rest on clinical or impressionistic methods. This naturally leads to a consideration of alternative interpretive strategies and the comparative accuracy they achieve.

Advantages of formal decision methods. Many general psychology texts describe the explanation, control, and prediction of behavior as among the great scientific goals of the field. Ironically, how best to achieve the predictive aim may have the clearest answer at this time, and yet this potentially invaluable knowledge is commonly overlooked or disregarded without sufficient consideration of the evidence. The succinct answer is that at present, across a wide array of areas in psychology, the prediction of outcomes or conditions is best accomplished overall through the use of formalized (statistical, actuarial) procedures for combining information. It is highly likely that the same applies to conclusions about malingering. This does not mean that subjective clinical judgment cannot attain a certain level of success or sometimes match statistical procedures, but only that when there is a difference between the two approaches actuarially based decisions are very likely to be more accurate, thus making it a superior method overall.

Terminology in this area is frequently confused or used idiosyncratically. Meehl (1954/1996) distinguished between *modes of data combination*—using either clinical judgment or established actuarial formulae—and the *kinds of data* relied on, which might be either objective (e.g., test scores) or subjective (e.g., clinical impressions from an interview). Confusion has been common in neuropsychology, where using actuarial procedures for combining data may be conflated with objective data entering into the combination. The fundamental issue here involves methods of data combination or interpretation, not the type of data that are combined. Another source of confusion has been to equate merely automated or structured methods for data combination (e.g., computerized interpretation) with a truly actuarial method. With clinical (subjective) judgment methods, the professional combines and processes information in the head; with actuarial methods, the judge is excluded and instead data combination rests on two conjoint elements: (a) predetermined decision procedures that are (b) based on empirically established relations.

The two different methods of data combination can be illustrated by contrasting approaches to the evaluation of baseball players. A first scout uses clinical judgment. She obtains background information about characteristics such as height and weight, running speed, strength, and eye–hand coordination. Some of the information that enters into her decision-making may be objective (e.g., height), and other information may be subjective (e.g., effort, openness to coaching). Again, the kind of information upon which decisions are based needs to be distinguished from the type of method used to combine and interpret the data. This scout uses her judgment to appraise the players and formulate predictions about their future successes, using her background experience and knowledge to reach these decisions. She may consider more formal statistical information about baseball and baseball success, but she interprets and combines this information in her head. The second scout takes exactly the same information and enters it into a formula derived from empirically verified relations between status on these variables and baseball performance. When the actuarial (statistical) method is used, the *interpretive* process occurs independently of the scout; the formula (algorithm) determines the prospect's rating. To summarize the differences, with clinical judgment data are combined or interpreted in the head. With statistical methods data combination is formalized and based on established empirical relations. Note that with the latter, both conditions must be met to consider a method truly actuarial.

The mere fact that a computer is used does not necessarily mean that a method is actuarial because the dual requirements of a set decision procedure and interpretation based on empirically established relations must both be satisfied. Many computer-based test interpretations are not actuarial and rather are programmed to replicate a clinician's judgments. For example, a clinician might interpret a certain pattern of Minnesota Multiphasic Personality Inventory-2 (MMPI-2) scores as signaling a certain condition based on experience with the measure. If the computer is programmed to copy these judgments, but the judgments themselves are not based on empirically established relations or decision rules, then it is not employing an actuarial procedure. Arguments about the merits of computer-based interpretation in neuropsychology have often failed to distinguish between *automated* methods and *actuarial* methods. In these debates, the contrast really being discussed is clinical versus automated procedures, not clinical versus actuarial procedures, the latter of which often produces different results (a clear overall advantage for the actuarial method, as will be discussed below).

Nearly any form of judgment or prediction clinicians make can also be made, in theory, with actuarial methods (although this does not mean that judgmental accuracy will necessarily be equal overall, as will be described). It is a common misconception that only test data or objective data are amenable to actuarial methods. Actuarial methods do require some type of coding or quantification, but almost any form of qualitative information can be transformed into a useable format. For example, a test technician's subjective impression about level of effort can be rated, or the red flags frequently cited as tip-offs for malingering can be codified in some manner (e.g., 1 = present, 0 = absent). Just like many fruitless debates about qualitative versus quantitative data in neuropsychological assessment that rest on assumptions of exclusivity, this issue is minimally concerning because qualitative information or impressions are almost always quantifiable.

We have described pure forms of clinical and actuarial methods, but the methods may be blended to an extent in certain ways. For example, when appraising malingering, a neuropsychologist who ultimately combines information in her head may have conducted one or more actuarial analyses and have those results in mind when reaching conclusions. A major potential limit of such a "clinical-actuarial" approach is that in a sizeable percentage of cases the clinical and actuarial methods generate directly conflicting outcomes (e.g., brain damaged versus not brain damaged). Thus the notion sometimes voiced that clinical and actuarial methods can be combined seamlessly or that there is no inherent conflict between the two is inherently mistaken.

Research comparing clinical and statistical procedures. There have now been hundreds of studies conducted across more than 5 decades comparing clinical and actuarial methods. The majority of these studies involved mental health practitioners and cover a broad array of diagnostic and predictive tasks, neuropsychological assessment included in a limited number of instances. Meehl (1984) summarized research findings at that time as follows:

> It is safe to say... that the mass and qualitative variety of investigations of the predictive accuracy of subjective impressionistic human judgment, such as that exercised by the individual clinician or case conference or psychiatric team, versus that of even a crude non-optimized mechanical prediction function (equation, nomograph, actuarial table) is about as clearly decided in favor of the latter predictive mode as we can ever expect to get in the social sciences. *I am unaware of any other controversial matter in psychology for which the evidence is now so massive and almost 100% consistent in pointing in the same direction.* (p. xii)

Of interest, in an earlier review, Sawyer (1966) found that when data are interpreted clinically, less accurate conclusions are reached overall when interview data are added to test data. (We would caution the reader that Sawyer's analysis was limited to unstructured interview methods and does not necessarily apply, or apply equally, to structured interview methods.) Grove et al.'s (2000) meta-analysis similarly showed that adding interview data to other data led to an overall *decrease* in accuracy *when interpreted via clinical judgment*. In contrast, actuarial methods achieved greater overall accuracy when both interview and test data were available. The increase in accuracy attained when interview data are added to test data and interpreted via the actuarial method shows that interviews can or do generate useful information. However, when these two data sources are interpreted clinically, practitioners have difficulty separating more valuable information from less valuable or even invalid predictors.

Dawes et al.'s (1989) review also covered naturalistic studies in which clinicians were allowed to collect the data that they wanted in the manner they preferred. Dawes et al. found that these types of studies yielded outcomes parallel to other research on clinical versus actuarial methods, and further that simple actuarial formulae utilizing only a few variables also equaled or exceeded the accuracy of clinical judgment. One of the factors that Dawes et al. discuss underlying the overall superiority of actuarial methods is consistency (i.e., the same data always produce the same conclusion). Decision makers show random fluctuation in judgment, which decreases reliability and consequently the validity or accuracy of decision making.

Grove et al.'s (2000) meta-analysis included studies covering psychology and other fields (e.g., medicine). They found that actuarial methods were superior overall to clinical methods. The methods did tie in a considerable number of comparisons, but when there was a difference, the actuarial method was superior to the clinical method in the vast majority of instances. Clinicians' level of training or experience did not alter the overall actuarial advantage. Ægisdóttir et al.'s (2006) meta-analysis focused solely on the mental health field and included research that was unavailable when Grove et al. performed their work. The studies covered such diverse domains as psychiatric diagnosis, length of treatment, prognosis, suicide attempts, and neuropsychological assessment. They also found an overall advantage for the actuarial method over the clinical method, one that was slightly larger than Grove et al. reported.

The relative advantage of the actuarial method over the clinical method and the potential for reducing error becomes more palpable when placed in tabular form. Table 3 shows accuracy rates for all of the studies in the Ægisdóttir et al. meta-analysis that provided data on hit rates. Some studies did not provide this information, and thus the table includes most, but not all of the studies from their meta-analysis. For the highest level of accuracy shown, which might be considered good-to-excellent, the actuarial method achieved six to seven times the number of results in that range. Furthermore, the clinical method generated about twice as many results in the lowest category, which might be classified as weak or poor accuracy (as some of these results fall near or below chance level).

Viewed in absolute terms, assume that actuarial methods reduce total error rates on average by about 10–15%. This may represent the difference between an error rate of, say, 30–35% versus 20%, which is a very impressive and meaningful improvement. (Stated conversely, it represents an improvement in accuracy rates from about 65–70% to about 80%.) For example, if a neuropsychologist evaluated 2000 cases over a 10-year period, use of actuarial decision procedures could avoid 200–300 errors. Should the same hold in the area of malingering assessment—and there are strong reasons to believe it does (see below)—the common advice to rely primarily on clinical judgment would increase rather than decrease error and partly or fully negate the potential advantages of the methods so many have labored so hard to create. It is thus worth examining the topic of countervailing validated decision procedures.

Identifying exceptions to actuarial predictions. The issue of countervailing actuarial outcomes is germane for a number of reasons. Actuarial methods are certainly fallible and sometimes produce relatively high error rates. Hence, there are compelling reasons to try to do better. (What may be less acknowledged is that *the same concern applies as much or more to clinical methods* because they lead to more

Table 3 Summary of accuracy rates across studies for which Ægisdóttir et al. (2006) provided hit rates

Level of accuracy	Percentage of studies	
	Clinical method[a]	Actuarial method
.80–.99	3%	20%
.60–.79	60%	61%
.59 or less	38%	19%

[a]Percentages sum to more than 100 due to rounding error.

frequent error overall than actuarial methods.) Similarly, circumstances arise that seem to argue for the rejection of actuarial predictions. For example, suppose a method for malingering detection that depends on the contrast between expected and obtained levels of performance is administered to someone with a mild head injury. This individual obtains a score slightly beyond the cutoff for identifying insufficient effort but also presents with a sleep disorder and may be experiencing medication side effects. The matter of countervailing is also of particular interest because the simple reality is that clinicians often do freely countervail or disregard actuarial outcomes (e.g., see Hanson & Morton-Bourgon, 2009; Ruscio, 2003). Thus, it is critical to examine the results of such common judgmental practices and compare them to more consistent reliance on actuarial methods.

There are certainly many instances in which clinical conclusions conflict with the outcomes that would be reached using actuarial methods, but there is a lack of awareness or concern about actuarial methods. When actuarial outcomes are known but rejected, commonly cited reasons are that the actuarial method does not apply to the case at hand or to the clinician herself. In essence, the clinician assumes she knows best when to accept or not accept the actuarial outcome, and that by exercising this sort of discretion she can exceed or bolster the accuracy of actuarial methods.

Although there is insufficient literature on this topic to draw strong conclusions, most of the studies do not support such decision policies (e.g., Grove et al., 2000; Hanson & Morton-Bourgon, 2009; Leli & Filskov, 1981; Sawyer, 1966). Sawyer identified a few studies in which clinicians were provided with the outcome of actuarial analyses and could use or disregard them at their discretion. The studies all showed that attempts at selective countervailing were unsuccessful and that the highest level of overall accuracy is achieved when clinicians consistently adhere to the actuarial method. Leli and Filskov (1981), in their study on the identification of brain damage and associated features, obtained the same basic outcome. More broadly, many studies comparing clinical and actuarial methods did provide clinicians with such information as test scores for which there is background research on actuarial or statistical analyses, and which they could use or disregard. These studies thus provide suggestive information on the success accomplished by following or countervailing actuarial outcomes at one's discretion versus following actuarial outcomes uniformly (i.e., the actuarial methods in the research). If a strategy of freely countervailing actuarial outcomes was successful, clinicians would be beating actuarial methods regularly or at least in a considerable minority of the cases, which clearly has not been the case (although for a rare and interesting exception within neuropsychology, but one limited to a single practitioner, see Fargo, Schefft,

Szaflarski, Howe, Yeh, & Privitera, 2008). Commenting more generally on this matter, Grove and Lloyd (2006) put the issue this way:

> As Paul [Meehl] pointed out, there may well be reasoning processes that clinicians sometimes use that a formula, table, or computer program cannot precisely mimic. However, whether such reasoning actually helps clinicians dependably outperform statistical formulas and computer programs is an empirical question with a clear, convincing answer: No, for prediction domains thus far studied. The burden of proof is now squarely on clinicians' shoulders to show, for new or existing prediction problems, that they can surpass simple statistical methods in accurately predicting human behavior. (p. 194)

Rather than embracing actuarial methods and the advantages that they provide in increasing judgmental accuracy, questionable reasons are sometimes given for dismissing this extensive body of evidence. A common argument is that all individuals are different and thus a general decision rule will necessarily prove ineffective. Such a position, despite its possible appeal, contradicts rudimentary principles of logic and rationality. For example, if an actuarial procedure for malingering detection achieves an 80% accuracy rate and is used with 100 individuals, on average it will identify 80 of those individuals correctly despite their uniqueness. This success is achieved because individuals may have elements in common, much like favoring chocolate ice cream over lima beans or preferring the news that the IRS was mistaken about a large penalty and a refund is on the way rather than the reverse.

The main issue is not realizing that exceptions occur, which is obvious from the success actuarial methods do and do not achieve, but identifying their occurrence, which is another matter. If identifying exceptions were easy, then as noted clinicians in the comparison studies would have beaten actuarial methods regularly, which certainly has not occurred. It is a simple matter of mathematics, not philosophy, that in those studies, for each erroneous actuarial outcome clinicians correct, there is at least one, and often more than one, correct actuarial outcome that is mistakenly overturned. Given the overall superiority of actuarial methods, a tally of all clinicians' countervails across all studies on the topic would show that considerably more have been wrong than right.

A genuine issue, not a pseudo-issue. Some have argued that the debate over clinical versus actuarial methods is fallacious or ill-conceived, that there is no true conflict between the two ways of proceeding and that they can be readily combined. Meehl's (1986) rejoinder exposes the fallacy of this thinking:

> Some critics asked a question... which I confess I am totally unable to understand: Why should Sarbin and Meehl be fomenting this needless controversy? Let me state as loudly and as clearly as I can manage, even if it distresses people who fear disagreement, that Sarbin and I did not artificially concoct a controversy or foment a needless fracas between two methods that complement each other and work together harmoniously. I think this is a ridiculous position when the context is the pragmatic context of decision making. You have two quite different procedures for combining a finite set of information to arrive at a predictive decision. It is obvious from the armchair, even if the data did not show it overwhelmingly, that the results of applying these two different techniques to the same data set do not always agree. On the contrary, they disagree a sizable fraction of the time. Now if a four-variable regression equation or a Glueck actuarial table tells the criminal court judge that this particular delinquent will probably commit another felony in the next 3 years and if a

case conference or a social worker says that he will probably not, it is absurd to say that Sarbin and I have "fomented a controversy" about how the judge should proceed. The plain fact is that he cannot act in accordance with both of these incompatible predictions. (p. 372)

Application to malingering assessment. There are strong grounds to believe that the same basic findings from the substantial literature on clinical versus actuarial methods apply similarly to neuropsychology and malingering assessment. It should be emphasized that this is a relative or comparative exercise and not a commentary on the accuracy or worth of neuropsychological assessment. How well neuropsychologists perform when interpreting data clinically is distinguishable from how they compare to actuarial methods. For example, Garb and Schramke's (1996) review suggests that in some situations clinical judgment in neuropsychology achieves about 85% accuracy (although accuracy rates on other tasks, such as localization of brain damage, appraisal of less gross or severe cases, differentiation of static versus progressive conditions, and malingering detection may be lower, and perhaps at times considerably so). An accuracy rate of 85% is certainly something in which to take pride, but knowing this or other rates for clinical judgment does not answer the question of whether we can do as well or better with actuarial methods. Furthermore, whichever method is most accurate, to the extent it performs well it remains a credit to the profession. It is no less commendable if, for some important task, psychologists or neuropsychologists have developed an actuarial method that improves on clinical judgment and further enhances human welfare.

Although research on this issue in neuropsychology is somewhat limited, trends observed in the general literature on clinical versus actuarial methods are also found in studies on neuropsychological assessment (Ægisdóttir et al., 2006; Grove et al., 2000), with an aforementioned notable exception being Fargo et al. (2008). The limited comparative research on clinical versus actuarial methods in malingering detection similarly reflects trends seen in the general literature. If in area after area in which comparative studies have been conducted, the actuarial method proves superior overall, what are the odds that matters would turn out differently in the specific area of malingering assessment? Surely, given the amount and range of research presently available, those odds are rather poor and one assuming exemption would seem to bear the burden of proof.

A neuropsychologist's sincere belief that she can beat the accuracy of actuarial procedures by countervailing their outcomes when it seems indicated is likely to lack formal evidence supporting the impression. An assertion such as, "Based on my clinical experience, I think that I achieve the best results by integrating all of the information and relying on my own clinical experience," obviously does not comprise scientific evidence and is unsubstantiated. The literature on the pervasiveness of overconfidence should also give us pause. One advantage of a properly developed actuarial method is that, in comparison to an unverified subjective impression, it generates information about how well it does and does not perform.

Implications of the comparative literature. The practical and scientific implications of research on data integration and clinical versus actuarial methods can now be examined. First, it is often counterproductive to try to use all of the data. When weak predictors are added to stronger predictors, they often decrease overall accuracy. If there is insufficient scientific evidence to make a reasonably trustworthy determination about level of validity for a measure or procedure (and especially if there are viable and well-established alternatives), there is rarely sufficient justification to include that questionable method. The quality of measures varies a great deal, and some are highly susceptible to error. When bad measures are combined with good measures, one is not adding information that increases the likelihood of a correct conclusion. Rather, one is adding weaker or poorer information to stronger information and, therefore, is much more likely to increase the chances of error. If a weak measure yields the same result as superior measures, it changes little or nothing. If it is in disagreement, it will most likely be wrong, and the less accurate a measure the more likely it is to yield different results than accurate measures.

Second, adding redundant predictors often does little or nothing to increase accuracy, especially as the level of redundancy increases. A second measure that is highly correlated with a first measure will give us little additional predictive punch. In general, we should seek predictors that are maximally valid and minimally redundant with one another.

Third, for specific predictive tasks, we often approach or reach a ceiling in accuracy once we have properly combined our two, or three, or perhaps four or five best, minimally redundant predictors. If we have even a relatively small set of such predictors, we should be conservative about adding further variables.

Fourth, as each of the preceding points suggests, incremental validity usually should be the key criterion in deciding whether to include information in data gathering or interpretive procedures. Even if a measure has validity, this in itself does not ensure a contribution to incremental validity. Furthermore, incremental validity is unlikely to be achieved when a weak predictor (and obviously an invalid one) is combined with a strong predictor or predictors, making survey results suggesting continued heavy reliance on subjective and even unverified methods in comparison to methods with stronger scientific support a clear concern.

Fifth, it would help to become less enamored with complex pattern analysis, especially to the extent that extreme and unyielding commitment to such approaches leads to underuse or neglect of alternative procedures that are more likely to enhance accuracy. (Simpler types of pattern analysis are far more viable, and our cautions here focus on the more complex forms of analysis that are often advocated.) The vast literature on clinical versus actuarial methods offers a compelling demonstration that given our current state of knowledge, and despite the many important advances in our field, maximizing predictive accuracy does not necessarily require complex pattern analysis. Many statistical prediction procedures are exercises in simplification, but simplification that works (given our current state of knowledge) as well as or better than efforts at complex data integration. For example, an actuarial method for malingering detection may divide individuals across a couple of variables, merely add up a few scores without considering interrelations, and then apply a dichotomous cutoff score. The reasons attempts at *complex* pattern analysis often fall short were touched on and will not be reiterated here, although we will note that perhaps the biggest obstacle is the poor reliability of the so-called patterns that neuropsychological data often produce. One of the current authors describes more than half a dozen powerful factors that are frequently present in psychological and neuropsychological data that distort test score patterns (Faust, in preparation). Although these factors create different sorts of influences, for most the final common impact is to erode, often to an extreme degree, the reliability and validity of obtained patterns.

Sixth, researchers in psychology and neuropsychology have done a remarkable job developing formal methods for assessing malingering and developing other helpful decision procedures. We should make good use of these measures and be cautious about too quickly or freely countervailing actuarial outcomes. Consistent with the work of Arkes and others (Arkes, 1981; Arkes, Dawes, & Christensen, 1986; Sieck & Arkes, 2005), it may be productive if decision makers deliberately generate explicit reasons an actuarial outcome might be accurate and a competing decision they currently favor might be inaccurate before rejecting the former. Generating reasons for an alternative outcome tends to make evidence contrary to one's initial conclusions more salient and can reduce unjustified levels of confidence. When levels of confidence in impressionistic judgment become more realistic, the comparative merits or potential superiority of actuarial statistical rules may become more evident and compelling.

The above considerations spell out certain critical research needs. Given the number of malingering indicators we now have that have been supported through research, it would be helpful to examine indicators that have not been studied adequately but that still seem to be used frequently in clinical practice. Frequency of use could easily be identified through surveys. Examining these indicators might add to the pool of validated methods and, of equal importance, help us to identify those variables we have been using that are not valid or are weaker than other alternatives.

There is limited utility in identifying or developing indicators that are redundant with previously available ones. Rather, there is more to gain by trying to uncover variables that are likely to contribute unique predictive variance. This might be achieved by seeking new classes of predictors (see further below). It would also be beneficial if a greater effort was made to assess incremental validity. Many studies involve single predictors or a few predictors. Although there is nothing wrong with this per se, we need to take the next step and examine incremental validity more fully. Given the number of malingering indicators that are now available, one could argue that a study limited to showing that a new variable has discriminating power is of negligible help because we cannot evaluate whether that variable will have a negative, positive, or neutral effect on predictive accuracy when combined with other variables.

Although there has been some increase in attention to incremental validity in recent years that we will detail later, there are still considerable gaps in knowledge. Even acknowledging these limits, as well as limits in the literature comparing clinical and actuarial judgment in neuropsychology, we can still go a long way toward applying the existent knowledge and derived principles in these areas. Some investigators have examined multiple variables and their combined effects, which is a start; but some of these studies do not go far beyond adding to the growing number of demonstrations of a matter that is not in question—that the statistical combination of multiple valid predictors will usually outperform a single valid predictor. What these studies do not examine is the effect of combining new predictors with the best available predictors. Although comprehensive studies of incremental validity are often lacking in malingering detection, there are quite a few studies examining combinations of variables. Other research looks at correlations among such variables, and such studies can help inform us about their degree of redundancy. For example, we may find that three variables have similar levels of validity, and that the first variable is highly correlated with the second variable but only modestly associated with the third variable. This suggests that the combination of the first and third variables should produce greater accuracy than the combination of the first two variables; the first and second variables are redundant, but the third variable adds unique predictive variance. Likewise, studies addressing the impact of combining variables, even if not comprehensive, provide a good start in making educated selections and formulating judgments about their joint properties. Although even limited formal information about combined variables and a conservative approach to incorporating variables into formulations may well work better than impressionistic methods that attempt to integrate large amounts of information, it is not a given and certainly should be appraised through formal research.

Availability of validated decision methods. Despite what may be common belief, actuarial procedures or statistical decision methods are not sparse in neuropsychology and malingering detection. There is a broad tendency to conflate: a) comparative studies on clinical versus statistical methods with b) the availability of statistical or actuarial decision procedures. Across psychology, there are *hundreds* of studies comparing clinical and actuarial methods but *thousands* of studies on the development and evaluation of statistical decision procedures. Similarly, there are now hundreds of studies on statistical or actuarial methods for malingering detection. As described, the many comparative studies show that with rare exception, actuarial procedures equal or exceed clinical judgment and thus are superior overall. Given this extensive and consistent background research and the diversity of areas that have been covered, the likelihood that properly developed actuarial methods will turn out to equal or surpass clinical judgment in a domain not yet adequately studied, including malingering detection, is high or very high.

The potential value of expanding the already considerable body of *comparative* literature on clinical versus actuarial judgment to other areas of clinical relevance, however, is a distinct issue from the availability of statistical and actuarial methods themselves. Further, to argue that we should default to the decision-making approach that is inferior overall (i.e., clinical judgment) because we lack a comparative study specific to the task we are undertaking is almost certainly less justifiable than the alternative position or choice (i.e., to depend instead on the method that research has almost always shown to be as good or better).

The development of actuarial methods will be partly bound by our overall knowledge of malingering. It is often easiest to develop highly accurate actuarial procedures where we least need them, such as methods that merely distinguish normal individuals doing their best versus those simulating poor performance. However, it is a serious philosophical error to believe that one needs a gold standard or nearly infallible criteria to develop useful knowledge and decision rules, for were this the case, much of science could never have progressed. What if Galileo had concluded that peering through the telescope was useless because he had no final authority to test the accuracy of his observations? It can be difficult, but not impossible, to develop useful actuarial methods for malingering detection absent a highly accurate method for identifying its presence, as we will take up at length in the section directed toward research needs. One major theme of the current work is that there are many ways to push the boundaries of knowledge, even when we do not have information that would seem crucial to the task. It is particularly encouraging that in a number of areas in which concentrated efforts have been made to refine actuarial methods (especially within the forensic arena), accuracy seems to have grown steadily (see Faust & Ahern, 2011), and there is good reason to believe that these positive trends will continue within neuropsychology and malingering detection.

Failure to Consider or Properly Apply Base Rates

A *base rate* refers to the frequency of occurrence, whether the subject matter is the number of bee bites in the United States annually, how often it rains in the Sonoran Desert, or the number of individuals who sustain mild head injuries within a certain population. Base rates are among the most useful aids in diagnosis and predication and sometimes by themselves are, far and away, the single most powerful diagnostic or predictive indicator. Acquisition of more refined knowledge about base rates and proper utilization of that information can improve accuracy remarkably, thereby serving to advance some of our most worthy goals and meriting a high position in our profession's priority list. As this section of the current work addresses interpretive methods, applied issues in the use of base rates will be addressed here, with research needs and suggestions discussed subsequently. It is surely evident that research knowledge about base rates and application go hand in hand because application cannot be better than the knowledge on which it depends. At the same time, certain problems in the application of base rates do not start with limitations in research knowledge but with what might be considered misguided advice. As will be discussed, some suggestions for the use of base rates in malingering detection are most likely to degrade or reverse potential benefits.

Various studies demonstrate the underuse or neglect of base rates (e.g., Gouvier, 2001; Kennedy, Willis, & Faust, 1997; Labarge, McCaffrey, & Brown, 2003; Nickerson, 2004). Nickerson observed that base rates are often underweighted or disregarded, and that case-specific information often impedes their use. Case-specific information refers to almost any detail about an individual. For example, if only base rate information is available (e.g., 15% of children in a certain school setting have attention-deficit/hyperactivity disorder), that information may well be used properly. However, when specifics are added, even if they have no true diagnostic or predictive value, such individuating information activates associations or cognitive schema that distract attention from base rates (see Kennedy et al., 1997). Obviously, case-specific information will be available in virtually any forensic case in neuropsychology. The problem is not with the use of case-specific information per se, which of course may be highly relevant, but rather that such information, and even items of negligible value, can lead to underuse or neglect of base rates. Failure to persist on a few difficult items, which may be about as common among malingerers as among those with a certain neurological disorder and appear almost exactly alike behaviorally, may nevertheless strike the examiner in a certain way and be weighted as or more heavily than base rates for malingering in the setting. Such salient information, knowingly or unknowingly, can have an undue influence on conclusions.

Other research suggests that neuropsychologists may have difficulty using base rates properly. Labarge et al. (2003) found that most of the neuropsychologists in their study answered simple questions about base rates correctly but that a large percentage had difficulties when required to combine information about base rates with the diagnostic accuracy of clinical indicators or signs. In many situations (as will be discussed), unless both types of information are combined properly, clinicians are far more prone to error. The authors stated:

> Whether wittingly or unwittingly, the principle that the diagnostic utility of a sign is relative to the base rate of the disorder in question impacts the likelihood of accuracy of every test interpretation or diagnosis a neuropsychologist makes. Despite this fact, the majority of the neuropsychologists in the present study either neglected or misused base rate information when that information was presented explicitly in a format similar to that in which neuropsychologists would be expected to encounter it (i.e., as in the probability format). (p. 170)

On a positive note, Labarge et al. also found that presenting information in a more user-friendly format had a corrective influence, although about one-third of the neuropsychologists still did not perform adequately. Taken together, research suggests that base rates are commonly neglected, underweighted, or not applied properly or optimally, but also that improved practices are attainable through various means (see also Faust & Ahern, 2011). It is thus worthwhile to overview the application of base rates to malingering detection in neuropsychology.

Use of base rates to assist in dichotomous decisions. When considering the use of base rates, it is helpful to make certain key distinctions. The first is whether one faces a dichotomous decision task (e.g., hospitalize or do not hospitalize, malingering or not malingering) or, instead, is mainly interested in determining the likelihood of a condition or outcome (e.g., how likely it is that someone is malingering), because the two call for somewhat differing approaches. Also, certain additional adjustments need to be made when the determination of interest involves more than one condition (as is usually true when assessing malingering) and those conditions are not mutually exclusive but may co-occur (e.g., brain injured and malingering). It is easier to start with the simpler circumstance of dichotomous choices and then proceed to more complex determinations.

Suppose the dichotomous choice at issue is whether or not a criminal defendant is feigning severe cognitive compromise due to brain injury. For the moment we will assume that the benefits of a correct decision and the costs of an erroneous decision are about equal. In most such situations, the primary goal is simply to maximize decision accuracy. (If costs and benefits were uneven, we would likely have greater interest in reducing one or the other type of error, even if the end result reduced overall accuracy to some extent.)

Given a dichotomous decision, random selection results in an overall accuracy of 50%, which equates to the worst outcome obtained by following base rates uniformly when the choice is limited to two possibilities. It would be equivalent to letting a coin flip determine the decision. As the possibilities depart from 50%, there is a corresponding increase in the accuracy achieved by uniformly playing the base rates. If in the setting of interest condition A is present 80% of the time (and hence not-A occurs 20% of the time), assuming condition A every time yields an overall accuracy of 80%. In contrast, if an adolescent fails to apologize 80% of the time he is rude, then guessing that no apology will occur produces an overall accuracy rate of 80%. Here, non-occurrence is the more frequent "outcome" or behavior, and thus one playing the base rates predicts the behavior will *not* take place.

When frequency of occurrence is either very high or very low, uniformly adhering to the base rate produces extremely high accuracy rates. How often this situation applies in malingering assessment is uncertain and can depend a great deal on whether one counts nearly any instance of nonoptimal effort (in which case the identification may be of minimal value) or adopts a more stringent standard. It is certainly possible that in some treatment settings frequencies of unabashed malingering are quite low, and thus one can commonly achieve high accuracy rates by simply following the base rates. Broad recognition of such possibilities in treatment settings, along with other considerations, such as cost-benefit analysis of correct and incorrect identifications, are major reasons for adopting conservative approaches in such circumstances. At the same time, even when base rates achieve impressive levels of accuracy, unwavering and blind adherence to them in clinical or forensic practice can be perilous and usually is not advisable.

Assume now we have access to both a base rate and to one or another sign or indicator, such as the score on an effort test. The base rate and the test score may concur. For example, the base rate for malingering in the setting may be 25% and the test score may fall below a cutoff for identifying malingering. When both the base rate and another indicator (in this case a test score) point in the same direction, one does not need to elevate one over the other. However, in other instances the two will not agree, as would be the case if the test score exceeded the cutoff. When the clinician faces a dichotomous choice and the two predictive variables oppose one another, they cannot be "integrated" or "synthesized"—one must be selected and the other rejected.

If a test score and the base rate conflict, and if the primary intent is to maximize overall accuracy, one should use whichever variable is more accurate. For example, if the test achieves 70% accuracy and following the base rate achieves 85% accuracy, one selects the base rate over the test (which will cut the overall error rate in half, or from 30% to 15%). As follows, a test or diagnostic indicator will not outperform the base rate unless its accuracy exceeds the frequency of the more common occurrence (or non-occurrence). For example, if a test is 80% accurate in identifying malingering and the base rate for malingering is 60% in the setting of application, conflicts between the two should be decided in favor of the test. However, if the base rate for malingering was greater than 80% or lower than 20%, then playing the base rates (by guessing "yes" in the first instance and "no" in the second instance) would exceed 80% accuracy and inconsistencies with the test's results should be settled by deferring to the base rates.

It is probably evident that in order to make determinations about which data source or variable to follow, one prefers quality information about both the properties or accuracy of the test and the applicable base rates, which is precisely why knowledge about base rates and their appropriate application is so critical. As the examples are also intended to illustrate, the success that tests (and other diagnostic and predictive indicators) achieve varies in relation to base rates in the setting of application. Consequently, a test's value cannot be properly evaluated without accounting for base rates. For example, if overall accuracy is the main concern, a malingering test that achieves a 70% accuracy rate would be useful in a circumstance in which malingering occurs 50% of the time (e.g., criminal defendants caught red-handed who, despite a modest history of maladjustment, are pleading legal insanity), but of no help (or worse) in a setting with a base rate of 2%. (The same fundamentals apply to a test's accuracy rate, which also changes as the base rates vary, as will be discussed.)

It also follows that it may well be better to *not* use a valid test when dichotomous choices are involved and following the base rates yields clearly superior accuracy. In many such circumstances, a test result that concurs with the base rate will not alter the decision, and a result that conflicts with the base rate should be rejected. Aside from being a waste of time and expense, there is no legitimate purpose served by administering a test that should not be permitted to change anything. Even should the test be valid, if allowed to alter decision-making in such circumstances, it will most likely *decrease* accuracy.

The same fundamentals apply when a base rate is being compared to a composite of test scores or other variables. For example, although a single variable might not beat the base rates, combining variables could enhance accuracy and thereby succeed in doing so. Although there is a marked tendency to overestimate the contributions made by adding variables, there are of course many instances in which a combination of predictors performs better than a single predictor. As discussed in the prior section, however, intuitive judgments about the advantages of adding variables can easily go astray. Both validity and redundancy need be accounted for when determining whether to combine variables or how many variables to include. The improvement in predictive accuracy when combining variables may be considerably less than assumed, and a ceiling in predictive success for a specific judgment is often reached with only a small collection of variables. For example, if the best predictor achieves 70% accuracy, adding the next most helpful predictor may shift that level only marginally (especially when cross-validation is examined), and a third variable minimally, if at all. Thus, to assume that many variables will make a large contribution, especially without formal evidence or analysis of that possibility, will often lead to erroneous conclusions about the superiority of composites to judgments founded on the base rates. Again, overconfidence is a pervasive and often destructive impediment to sound judgment practices.

Similar fundamental principles also apply when more than two distinctions are at issue. For example, if one is attempting to distinguish between malingering, brain injury, and depression (and treating the three as distinct for illustrative purposes), then utilizing the base rates dictates selection of the most frequent alternative. However, as the number of choices expands, extreme base rates (and hence high rates of accuracy playing the base rates) are less common. Unfortunately, the same also holds for other predictive variables, such as tests: As the number of viable outcomes or possibilities expands, the accuracy of methods is likely to decrease proportionately. (It is true that as the possibilities multiply, guessing that one or another outcome will *not* occur has an increasing probability of being correct. However, this is often a vacuous accomplishment because it does not permit one to identify what *will* occur. For example, if we are walking through a dark alley in an urban center, we might be able to predict with nearly 100% accuracy that we will not be attacked by a hippopotamus, but that would be of little help if a violent criminal happens to cross paths with us. Similarly, when a patient sees her family doctor, guessing that the presenting problem is not a small toe fracture contributes little or nothing to a positive identification of the condition that might be present.)

Use of base rates to estimate probabilities. In many clinical and forensic situations, we are not so much interested in dichotomous choices but rather in determining the likelihood of an outcome or of multiple potential outcomes. Using different methods, base rates can be applied to estimate the likelihood of an outcome, with the best results often achieved by combining them with other valid predictors, such as test results. Incorporation of base rates into predictive formulations may improve accuracy substantially and, in some instances, reduce error multifold.

Much as is the case with dichotomous decisions, base rates and other valid predictors may point in the same direction. For example, the base rate for malingering in the circumstances under consideration might be about 15% and a test may yield a result indicting a 75% probability of good effort (or a 25% probability of insufficient effort). When the base rate and another valid indicator agree with one another and the two have some degree of independence (are not overly or entirely redundant), the joint probability of a given outcome is *greater* than the level of the stronger predictor alone. For example, assume that in the setting of interest the base rate for malingering is 70%. Further assume that a test achieves an overall accuracy rate of 80% in identifying malingering and shows some independence from the base rate. If the test result indicates insufficient effort as well, then the joint likelihood of malingering, given the base rate and test result, exceeds 80%. Alternatively, if the base rate and the outcome of a test both indicate the absence of malingering (e.g., the base rate is 15% and the test yields a negative outcome), the probability of nonoccurrence is more extreme than the odds indicated by the more accurate predictor. At other times, the base rate and other predictive variables will point in *opposite* directions, in which case the joint likelihood is *less* extreme than the level indicated by the stronger predictor. For example, if the base rate for malingering was 15% and the test indicated a 55% likelihood of malingering, the joint probability would be higher than 15% (but lower than 55%).[4]

When the accuracy achieved using the base rates exceeds the accuracy of the test by a considerable margin, as would not be unusual in settings in which base rates are extreme (e.g., clinical settings in which frequencies of malingering are rather low), the probability indicated by the test score or other indicator needs to be adjusted considerably. For example, a 30% likelihood may need to be adjusted to a 10% likelihood, or reduced by a factor of three. The greater the difference in predictive accuracy achieved by the base rate versus the test or other predictive variable, the greater the change in the joint probability.

These adjustments in joint probability are not easy to perform subjectively and can be counter-intuitive, potentially resulting in substantial error. They are best determined using formal methods that are designed exactly for this task and relatively simple to apply (see Meehl & Rosen, 1955; Waller et al., 2006, Chap. 9). More generally, base rates and other types of diagnostic or predictive variables and indicators for appraising malingering are not necessarily competitors. Rather, they can be combined to achieve more accurate judgments about likelihood and thereby provide considerable help to neuropsychologists in this and other contexts.

Which base rate to use. There are often legitimate reasons to question the quality of base rate information about malingering, a topic to be taken up at some length in the subsequent section on research needs. For the moment, it might be noted that the availability and quality of base rate information seem to be improving and various affirmative steps can be taken to further enhance our knowledge. However, even if high-quality base rate information is or becomes available, maximizing its benefit depends on implementing certain steps or principles. The advantage of using formal methods to integrate base rate information with other predictive variables has already been discussed. Another crucial matter, which seems to be a common source of confusion, is determining which base rates to use. A general figure is often of limited utility or even counterproductive because base rates can differ so much across settings of application or within subgroups. For example, if one is predicting the likelihood of a violent criminal offense, the base rate of such behavior is quite different among the general population as opposed to a group of repeat offenders with ongoing substance abuse problems. Consequently, the general population base rate would lead one astray if the examinee was of the latter sort. Base rates for the general population are often not nearly as useful as base

---

[4]These examples are somewhat oversimplified and disregard atypical circumstances that may modify outcomes, usually to a minimal degree. However, such potential exceptions argue for the use of formal methods for examining the combination of base rates with diagnostic signs and indicators, as referenced later in this section. Additionally, it may strike the reader as odd to refer to redundancy between diagnostic signs or tests and base rates, when there may seem to be a clear separation between the former two and base rates. The underlying basis for this reference to redundancy and the connection between tests signs or indicators and base rates is that signs and tests may achieve predictive power largely by association with differing base rates.

rates for population subgroups, making the identification of appropriate base rates critical in malingering detection.

The key here is to identify the base rate for the narrowest applicable group, with narrowness in this context defined by dimensions that: (a) alter the base rates and (b) are relevant to the individual under consideration. Suppose the examinee is undergoing neuropsychological assessment. Assume further that base rates for malingering differ in clinical and legal settings. Thus, if we know that the examinee is involved in litigation or being evaluated for this purpose, this characteristic is pertinent because it alters the base rates and is relevant to the individual. If one also knew that base rates for malingering varied between individuals with a certain cultural background versus another cultural background but this examinee came from neither background, the feature might alter base rates but would not be relevant to the examinee and thus would not help in narrowing the reference group. However, there may be other dimensions in addition to litigation status that also alter the base rates and are relevant, such as a prior history of questionable lawsuits. Other dimensions may be relevant but do not alter the base rates, such as demonstrations of apparent frustration during testing (a feature which may be similarly common among truly injured individuals and those feigning problems).

Although it might be assumed that numerous variables are needed to narrow down groups effectively, there is often much to be gained by identifying even one or a few pertinent dimensions because of the extent to which base rates can be impacted. Furthermore, for pragmatic and psychometric reasons, trying to extend the list beyond a limited set of variables often requires considerable effort yet produces rapidly diminishing gains. Such diminishing gains are especially likely to occur if one has already accounted for the variables that change the base rates the most (i.e., are maximally valid for their intended purpose) and are as non-overlapping (i.e., nonredundant) with each other as possible. Proceeding in this manner, a fairly small set of dimensions, often five or fewer, will approach or reach the ceiling in predictive utility, at which point further variables yield minimal or no improvement because of their redundancy. For example, both a history of multiple prior legal cases and certain psychological characteristics may be associated with a change in the base rates, but the two may occur together so frequently that only one of them needs to be used because the second adds almost no unique variance.

Recognizing flawed advice about the use of base rates. Some suggestions for narrowing down base rates are unsound. For example, according to one test manual, if about half of the cases seen in one's practice are forensic referrals, a certain assumed base rate for malingering might be used, and if the mixture differs the assumed rate should be modified. The recommendation partly follows from the reasonable supposition that base rates for malingering vary across clinical and forensic cases. However, it does not follow that one should try to derive an *overall* figure for one's setting based on the mix of clinical and forensic cases. This advice seems to reflect a serious misunderstanding about the use of base rates.

If one *cannot* determine whether examinees are being evaluated for clinical or legal purposes, then a composite base rate might be the best alternative, but of course one usually knows in advance (or at least when the evaluation is being conducted) whether litigation is involved. If the purpose of the evaluation can be ascertained, one should use the base rate for the applicable group. For instance, if one learns it is a clinical case and the assumed base rate for clinical cases is 5%, one uses that rate; and if one knows it is a legal case and the assumed base rate for legal cases is 20%, one uses this latter rate. If one instead followed the flawed advice to select a composite figure, it would increase the risk of false-positive errors for clinical cases (which is usually the mistake of greatest concern with patients) and the risk of false-negative errors for forensic cases. The problem with this composite strategy can be clearly illustrated if one assumes the identification of a progressive dementia is at issue and the average age of the neuropsychologist's referrals is 50, with a range from about 15 to 95 years. Certainly one would not use the base rate for that overall age group but rather the base rate that accords with the patient's age.

The need for subgroup norms, and the wide variation in malingering for different subgroups, is one reason why broad assertions about base rates are of limited value. Furthermore, given the current state of knowledge, base rate estimates sometimes can be markedly influenced by variations in the thresholds used to identify malingering. Perhaps most importantly, published estimates of base rates almost never address joint presentations (e.g., the frequency with which true injury and exaggeration co-occur), which we think is a vital matter and, when not accounted for, may produce highly misleading results. We will take up these and related matters when discussing major research needs.

With these cautions expressed, and acknowledging that the available data base for narrowing groups is commonly less complete than we would like, we should not overlook the meaningful gains in knowledge that have been achieved in various areas (e.g., see the discussion of post-concussion syndrome below). Narrowing the group along even one or two dimensions can augment the applicability and usefulness of base rates considerably. However, there are appropriate cautions and concerns about the quality of base rate information. For example, flaws in sampling methods or difficulties identifying representative samples may render such data of limited or questionable use. Nevertheless, as noted, increasing amounts of base rate data are available, and limitations in the quality of the information do not alter the basic principles underlying their use. Simply determining the range within which the base rates likely fall can sometimes be of considerable assistance, such as in circumstances in which conclusions do not change anywhere within that identified range. For example, even if one estimates the base rates for malingering to be as high as 50% in a certain setting, a negative result on a valid test is still likely to be correct. In the section on research applications, a number of suggestions are provided that may help to refine base rate estimates.

Use of base rates in covariation analysis. There is one other use of base rates that merits attention, which is in analyzing covariation or the association between variables. If there is a true association between a diagnostic sign or indicator and a condition or outcome, then that sign will occur more frequently when the condition is present than when it is absent (or, if it is a negative indicator, it will occur less frequently when the condition is present versus absent, the main point being its differential frequency). For example, if noncompliance with treatment is a valid indicator of malingering, then noncompliance should be more common among those who are versus those who are not malingering. Adopting the language of the current discussion, the base rate for the indicator should be higher in positive versus negative cases. It can thus be seen that basic covariation analysis requires frequency information about the occurrence of the diagnostic sign or indicator in a representative sample of positive and negative cases. Simply because something is frequent among a group of individuals with a certain condition does not necessarily mean it is a valid indicator of that condition, because it may occur at the same rate among those without the condition or those with various other conditions.

The ease with which characteristics that are frequent are potentially overperceived or misperceived as indicators of conditions is brought home in the previously described literature on illusory correlation, with a telling example in neuropsychology being research on potential signs of post-concussion syndrome (Gouvier, Cubic, Jones, Brantley, & Cutlip, 1992; Gouvier, Uddo-Crane, & Brown, 1988; Gunstad & Suhr, 2004; Iverson & Lange, 2003; Mittenberg et al., 1992; Wong, Regennitter, & Barris, 1994). For example, Gouvier et al. (1988) obtained few significant differences when comparing relatives' reports of various problems among a group of presumably normal college students to results obtained in studies of patients with mild to moderate head injuries. Even among the college students, high endorsement rates were observed on items addressing such features as memory disorder or changes in temper control. Subsequent studies produced similar outcomes (e.g., Gunstad & Suhl, 2004; Iverson & Lange, 2003), leading Iverson and Lange to warn that various characteristics often used to identify post-concussion syndrome are common among normal individuals. One certainly worries that some of the qualitative indicators or supposed signs that clinicians may rely on heavily to identify malingering (see Sharland & Gfeller, 2007) may be less valid than other indicators, or invalid, thereby degrading accuracy or leading to frequent errors. Considering the greater relative damage that can be caused by incorporating an invalid variable into clinical formulations (in comparison to omitting a valid one when other quality indicators are available), it is almost always worthwhile to ask whether the indicator at issue has, at minimum, been subjected to proper covariation analysis.

Misappraisal of Injury Severity

It is probably evident that methods for malingering detection and interpretive strategies may interact in a positive or negative manner (as is true as well for the examinee factors discussed below). For example, detection strategies that place heavy emphasis on pattern analysis are particularly susceptible to the inclusion of procedures with shaky reliability, and consequently if weaker variables are combined with stronger ones it may well diminish accuracy. With detection methods that compare performance to expected levels for the injury in question, overestimating injury severity will likely raise the frequency of false-negative errors and underestimating severity the rate of false-positive errors. Misappraisal of injury severity may be especially common when the neuropsychologist does not make sufficient effort to gather collateral information that is less susceptible to intentional distortion. For example, an individual who is purposely underperforming is probably also more likely to overdescribe an injury (e.g., asserting she was unconscious for a considerably longer period of time than was actually the case). Even should the neuropsychologist seek other records, they, too, may contain inaccuracies that the plaintiff promulgated. For example, a year earlier the plaintiff may have provided her primary doctor with the same misinformation; just because similar information is present in the previous record does not mean it is truly confirming. In contrast, it is not so easy to fake a cerebral bleed on an MRI. Additionally, independent informational sources, especially those more contemporaneous to the injury in question, may be helpful. If the ambulance run sheet describes the plaintiff as conversant and coherent 5 min after the event, it obviously is inconsistent with a report of extended loss of consciousness, whereas an inability to respond to first arrivers at the scene and take even simple steps to escape from a smoking vehicle would tend to corroborate initial confusion.

Some procedures that rely on performance below expected levels as the primary detection strategy frequently generate large differences between noncooperative individuals and those with moderate or even severe disorder. For example, a measure like the Test of Memory Malingering (Tombaugh, 1996) tends to achieve wide disparity between those with true injuries and those making insufficient effort. For other procedures, however, as disorder becomes more severe, overlap in performance levels may become substantial. Such overlap seems to occur most often when this detection strategy is used with standard tests, which typically are not designed to appear more difficult than they truly are. For example, scales from standard intelligence or memory tests often do not achieve marked separation between malingerers and those with moderate to severe brain injuries. Furthermore, if most individuals in the background research used to identify cutting points have experienced, say, mild brain injuries, but the plaintiff suffered a moderate-to-severe injury, then despite the plaintiff's best efforts her scores may not reach "expected" levels and misclassification as a falsifier may result. This issue becomes even more concerning and potentially confounded when these methods are used with individuals whose test performances may be suppressed by language or cultural factors or other potential inequities.

A serious error may also occur if a defense expert accepts the report of an individual who lacks insight given the magnitude of brain damage, obtains test scores below expectation for the severity of injury described, and consequently concludes the individual is a falsifier. Similarly, if methods are used that do not achieve particularly large separations between those putting forth inadequate effort and those with true injuries, the latter individuals, especially those who are also among the most unlucky (those who tend to experience the worst outcomes from their injuries), are at highest risk for false-positive identification.

4.6   Examinee Factors

In this section, we will discuss various examinee factors that can contribute to false-positive and false-negative errors. Coverage of examinee factors that appear in Table 1 will be selective because a number of the entries should be self-explanatory. At times we will touch on implications for research. However, when the research issues are more involved or seem to merit particular emphasis we will defer discussion to the next section on pressing investigative needs.

The Skill of the Falsifier

When appraising the generalization of research on malingering detection to genuine cases or one's practice, one of the most important and difficult issues to evaluate is representativeness. Studies involving malingerers who can be identified with relative ease due to extreme presentations are unlikely to mirror the distribution of cases seen in practice or to involve the kind of cases for which help is most needed. This concern would be resolved with relative ease if we could recruit truly representative samples of malingerers. The immediate barrier to doing so is that one would have to know how to identify malingerers before undertaking the investigations needed to learn how to identify malingerers—but if we possessed this knowledge, the studies would not be required in the first place. Such barriers are difficult but common in science, and they have usually proved surmountable with well-directed and persistent effort. Possible strategies for gathering representative samples will be discussed later. For the moment we wish to focus on one of the more important ways "real-life" malingerers might differ from subjects in studies, especially studies using extreme or obvious cases, this being level of skill.

Real malingerers may well be more skilled on average than typical research subjects, which can result in alterations in amount or kind, such as mean scores on quantitative indices or in the frequency with which certain so-called "red flags" are present. For example, delayed responding may be more common among research subjects instructed to lie because their misrepresentations may be far less practiced in comparison to habitual fabricators, especially when the latter have been given repeated opportunities to refine a story line for their legal cases.

Beyond concerns about the representativeness of research samples, there is a similar concern that malingerers in legal cases will show varying levels of proficiency, and that the higher the level of skill the greater the risk of false-negative error. This likelihood compounds the possibility that detection methods emerging from studies of more extreme cases may be ineffective with subgroups of malingerers that we are most interested in learning to detect more effectively. For example, whether in a research study or in forensic practice, it is not too difficult to identify someone who performs well below chance level on forced-choice methods and obtains abysmal scores nearly across the board. In forensic evaluations, the ease of detection will also be augmented if these test performances grossly misalign with other behaviors or reflections of functional capacity, such as the ability to converse normally and carry on various life activities without apparent difficulty. The less proficient the malingerer, the easier the detection task usually becomes. But in pushing the boundaries of our scientific knowhow and enhancing our overall capacity to differentiate between malingering and nonmalingering, increased study of more skilled malingerers is needed.

Investigations into skill levels could address the issue in multiple ways. It is highly unlikely that skill in malingering is restricted to those who do malinger, and, in any case, malingerers originate from the general population. As a result, it should not be difficult to create conditions in which skill can be assessed and its impact investigated. There are various fallible, but valid, measures of malingering. It is highly probable that the more of these measures an individual can circumvent the greater his skill in malingering, or at least the more difficult it will likely be to identify him correctly. Such an approach requires measures with some degree of independence, and conditions in which completing an earlier measure or measures does not markedly impact the effectiveness of subsequent measures used in the study, as might occur were a number of similar, forced-choice methods selected.

Suppose, for example, a researcher is evaluating the success of new procedure X in relation to skill level as defined by the ability to beat available measures. First, other measures of demonstrated validity can be administered and, based on the outcomes, subjects assigned a skill rating. Such studies need to be conducted anyway because they provide essential information about incremental validity and thus how to create effective or optimal composites of malingering measures. In a related or supplemental condition, one might have clinicians attempt to classify subjects. The frequency with which subjects beat the clinicians might enhance appraisal of subjects' skill ratings or at least provide a measure of the difficulty clinicians are likely to have with accurate identification.

Exact appraisals of skill are not necessary to make progress in such investigations. Although identification of skill level using these or other approaches will be imprecise, the main condition one needs to satisfy is a strong likelihood that the high-skill group is substantially more skilled than the low-skill group. If the researcher has a means for estimating the frequency of misclassification in group assignment, that is all the better. In many circumstances, all that is required are these contrasting (impure but different) groups to make progress with the needed forms of validation. Dawes and Meehl (1966) described methods and conditions under which validation work can proceed even when groups are far from pure, strategies that Jewsbury and Bowden (2014) have further explicated, and we will also discuss other possible research strategies in the next section.

Preparation/"Coaching"/Incentives

Many malingering tests are potentially susceptible to foreknowledge of their design, and very limited knowledge might often prove sufficient to escape detection. For example, merely knowing that if one is presented with two choices, one had better not perform below chance level may prove sufficient, especially given the high thresholds practitioners may set for identifying malingering.

How accessible is information about the design of malingering tests? Out of curiosity, one of the volume authors performed an internet search for a popular malingering test. The name of the test was entered, and the first resultant hit provided pictures of the manual and test booklets (which an examinee could then easily recognize), along with a brief and succinct explanation of the underlying detection strategy in easily understandable terms; the total time expenditure to find this information was under 60 s. Bauer and McCaffrey (2006) provided a considerably more detailed and formal examination of internet sources on malingering that should give almost any neuropsychologist involved in such matters an unsettled feeling. Additionally, various professional books are available online that offer detailed descriptions of malingering tests and detection strategies.

Kovach provided a striking and more direct example of the potential impact of coaching on effort tests, providing information about a forced-choice test that could be found with relative ease through an internet search (Kovach & Faust, in preparation). As Kovach pointed out, many coaching studies seem to have provided participants with information of limited utility, thereby potentially subjecting measures to insufficiently stringent examination of their susceptibility to coaching. In Kovach's study, brief but explicit information was provided about the design of the measure and a possible strategy for escaping detection. The effort test was embedded with standard memory measures, and participants were not provided with guidance about how to distinguish the effort test from the genuine measures. Limitations of the study included sample size and restriction to college students, but the results were uniform. Most of the participants in the fake-bad group underperformed on one or more of the genuine memory measures, but none of them "failed" the effort test: the false-negative rate was 100%.

Research also suggests that at least some lawyers warn litigants about malingering tests or might prepare them to complete the measures (Brennan, Meyer, David, Pella, Hill, & Gouvier, 2009). Whether this occurs or not, various other individuals may be able to provide coaching (e.g., test-wise prisoners in criminal cases) and, as noted, litigants may be able to obtain information about tests without much difficulty, especially in the age of the internet. As foreknowledge might make it fairly easy to beat certain effort tests, one obvious implication is that experts should consider using at least one measure that studies suggest is less susceptible to preparation or knowledge about its design, such as the Validity Indicator Profile (Frederick, 2003).

Another connected issue involves the magnitude of incentives in legal cases compared to those that might be offered in research studies. In legal cases, incentives may not be important so much for how they alter effort in the examination setting, but rather for what they lead individuals to do before they get there, and thus they relate in important ways to issues involving preparation and coaching. Someone who stands to gain lifetime financial security may spend considerable time preparing to malinger. For example, she may read extensively about the disorder she will fake and about psychological assessment instruments. Additionally, positive and negative incentives may impact greatly on the level of inconvenience, pain, and suffering an individual might be willing to tolerate in an effort to present a convincing picture. It is doubtful that the typical small rewards researchers offer would lead many individuals to load their bodies with anticonvulsants or submit to painful medical procedures. An individual who might avoid the electric chair by faking mental incompetence has a cost-benefit ledger from another universe.

Preparation would not seem too difficult a variable to study because the researcher can mimic and telescope experience. Two of the dimensions to be addressed are knowledge about (a) the disorder to be faked and (b) the strategies for malingering detection. The safest approach, or at least a means for testing the limits of methods, is to provide subjects with high-quality information about one or both dimensions (although a researcher might be interested in varying amounts or quality of information given). Fortunately, an increasing number of studies are examining the influence of knowledge on malingerers' success (e.g., Brennan et al., 2009; Cliffe, 1992; Frederick & Foster, 1991; Rogers, 2008; Rogers, Bagby, & Chakraborty, 1993; Wetter, Baer, Berry, & Reynolds, 1994).

There are very likely to be interactions between forms of knowledge and assessment methods. For example, although knowledge of a disorder might provide little aid in successfully altering an MMPI-2 profile, it might well be helpful in creating certain interview impressions. Someone with intimate knowledge about head injury, including features that fall outside general knowledge (e.g., "I've been seasoning my food a lot more"), would seem more likely than a naïve individual to fool an interviewer. This is one reason why studies examining general knowledge of disorder (what most people know even if they do not prepare themselves) are potentially so useful and can also inform the researcher about how much has to be done to mimic conditions of preparedness. Along these lines, because it is not necessarily done, researchers might make a systematic effort to assess baseline knowledge of subjects asked to malinger or who are about to be educated, and then, after providing information, check on understanding or mastery of the material. There is considerable value in furthering the development of methods that are less transparent or less susceptible to knowledge of strategy, lest even high-quality measures have a short half-life, a matter to be taken up in some detail in the section on research needs.

More generally, it is highly questionable how much incentives that are offered in studies (e.g., $10) bring investigators closer to real life. The positive incentives for malingering in real-life situations can be enormously larger; researchers can hardly afford to offer each successful subject a million dollars. Further, not all malingerers have positive incentives to falsify, and instead the primary motive may be to avoid something bad, such as a jail term. Additionally, whether or not positive incentives are present, there are almost always negative consequences for malingerers who fail (e.g., public exposure, debt). In a case in which one of the authors consulted, a lawyer claimed that because of neurocognitive deficits, he could no longer continue in what had been a successful practice. If he was malingering and if he lost his case, he would have been faced with financial disaster, for he probably could not have resumed his practice.

The potential of negative consequences, and sometimes severe ones, changes the dynamics of the situation. Powerful negative incentives may well alter who tries to malinger and may greatly magnify the intensity of the situation. As is well known, incentives may increase or decrease performance levels. In some circumstances, when motivation is extreme, effort is extreme but performance suffers, including perhaps the effectiveness of feigning. If a researcher's intent is mainly to increase compliance and effort, then manipulation checks may be as or more effective than typical incentives offered in studies.

Overlap and Other Factors Compromising Effort

At the risk of stating the obvious, in psychology and neuropsychology, many different things have common features or look alike. Such overlap often characterizes a range of elements that enter into judgments about cooperation with examination procedures, falsification, and other potential sources of inaccurate information. For example, an individual who suffers from cognitive dysfunction due to a past history of alcohol abuse but provides a false report that difficulties started at the time of the accident may display genuine disorder with features that overlap considerably with those one might see with head injury. Or, making things even more complex, that individual may also have experienced a prior (but unreported) head injury.

As the example illustrates, one or more co-occurring conditions, such as vascular disease, depression, or sleep apnea, are often present given their frequency among litigants. These additional conditions, which may be entirely independent of an injury or accident, can complicate the differential considerably. Further, such co-occurring conditions, when combined with the effects of an accident, may lead to performances that fall well below expected levels based on studies of the injury at issue. Such research, however, often excludes most or all subjects with these types of co-occurring conditions, and thus the results represent outcomes when the injury occurs in the absence of other factors that can diminish neuropsychological functioning and not when one or more of these other factors are also present. The consequence of overlap in presenting features and this gap between studies examining pure forms of injury and the additional complicating factors that are so common among plaintiffs is to magnify the risk of misidentifying malingering.

Thus far, much of the work on malingering detection in neuropsychology has been directed toward identifying *inadequate* effort. *Sufficient* effort is often identified by default, an approach with serious limitations. Level of effort certainly is not all or none, and many individuals whose effort would not be labeled grossly inadequate are, at the same time, not sustaining satisfactory or high levels of effort. Many organic and affective conditions can impede effort, and one consequence is often uneven or waning effort over time. Surely one of the most common consequences of serious brain injury is reduced endurance or difficulty sustaining effort. In many instances the level, consistency, and maintenance of effort are among the most important factors dictating what a patient can and cannot do and should be a target of treatment. In clinical settings, the most common cause of insufficient effort or failure to maintain adequate effort almost surely is not malingering but the primary or secondary effects of brain injury and affective disorder.

Fluctuations or Changes in Conditions

Some injuries or conditions usually improve over time, some get worse, and others tend to wax and wane. Lists of potential red flags for identifying malingering and formal approaches that appraise inconsistencies or decline in test performance may have value when expectations are for improvement or a steady course over time. Such methods can obviously be inappropriate or problematic when the true condition has been misidentified or when co-occurring conditions with uneven or progressive courses are superimposed on a correctly identified condition. For example, suppose the plaintiff initially experiences a head injury that, while improving over time, sets off a secondary depression that creates cycles of very poor functioning. If retesting happens to be conducted when the depression is at its worst, declining scores on measures of mental speed or visual learning may be mistaken for insufficient effort.

Alternatively, suppose the plaintiff did suffer a head injury in an accident and also has co-occurring conditions with entirely independent causes. Nevertheless, worsening of these independent conditions, such as diabetes and related vascular disease, may cause a decline in neuropsychological status that masquerades as malingering when methods are used that emphasize instability or decline in test performance. When clinical judgment is applied, fluctuations in co-occurring conditions, and hence in self-reports of symptoms and functional status, could be mistaken for attempts at falsification or difficulties remembering prior self-descriptions because they were fabricated. One could also see how an expert who is not particularly concerned with fairness could easily obtain a false-positive result on a malingering measure that could, nonetheless, be very difficult to uncover or correct without diligent effort. Although one may be disinclined to think that members of the profession would engage in such unscrupulous behavior, it would be unrealistic to believe it never happens. One protection is for those who develop methods for appraising effort to clearly point out limitations. To the credit of the profession, broad or general cautions are indeed often provided. However, more specific cautions that account for potential interactions between the detection strategy and situations in which it is vulnerable to error are not always offered and could provide an added level of protection against inappropriate applications.

Given the changes that can occur in conditions, a group of particular interest is those who were symptomatic, have largely or fully recovered, yet continue to describe or portray impairment. The experience of having been impaired might be highly informative for someone who wishes to feign disorder after recovery has taken place. The subsequent discussion covering potential co-occurrence of injury and exaggeration provides further material on this topic.

Complexity

Prior materials have already touched on this point to some extent, but to state it most directly, the more elements that are present that can influence the accuracy of information and the more possibilities the clinician must consider, then all else being equal, the more difficult the decision task. For example, some plaintiffs present with a history of multiple prior injuries and diseases that have yielded thousands of pages of prior records. They may seem to be unreliable historians, although to an uncertain extent genuine impairments may impede recollection or reporting capacities. On neuropsychological assessment, they may generate an unusual mix of results that raise various possibilities, and certain co-occurring conditions may create vexing alterations in test performance. For example, if a test is designed to appear more difficult than it really is, then not only individuals feigning disorder but also those who are exceedingly anxious or suggestible may underperform. Furthermore, if an individual with pronounced somaticizing tendencies falsely believes he has a serious head injury, the appearance of difficulty may lead to immediate discouragement and disengagement with a task and hence results that seem to reflect deliberate failure. It is clear that individuals who are genuinely injured *and* are also exaggerating or falsifying constitute a highly relevant and frequently occurring "mixed presentation" group that merits much greater investigation.

Less Well-Studied Conditions

The majority of malingering research involves closed head injury, especially mild to moderate head injury, which is understandable. These cases are common, are often the ones in which the presence of true injury will be most heavily contested, and regularly involve difficult differentiations. However, malingering research on mild to moderate closed head trauma may be of questionable applicability to cases that differ in amount or kind, such as more severe head trauma or other types of impairments or conditions. Further, there may be minimal research examining generalization of findings to different groups, and little investigation on the features that differentiate between individuals who truly suffer from these other injuries or conditions and those feigning such disorders. For example, we know far more about malingering of mild head injury than malingering in cases involving possible electrical trauma or exposure to such toxins as carbon monoxide, yet these and various other conditions are seen in litigation with some frequency.

Concerns about generalization are especially germane with approaches that depend on patterns of highs and lows or atypical performances. What is atypical for a mild closed head injury may be far more common, for example, with more localized injuries or injuries following exposure to solvents. Additionally, the same features that help separate falsifiers from those with genuine symptoms following a mild head injury may misidentify individuals with other types of genuine disorders or conditions as falsifiers. For example, mild head injury may create functionally significant reductions in new learning but rarely more than mild or moderate levels of impairment. Consequently, very low performance on tests tapping new learning may, instead, be suggestive of exaggeration or fabrication of deficit. In contrast, high-level carbon monoxide exposure may cause extreme impairments in new learning that frequently place individuals beyond cutoffs for malingering derived through studies of mild head injury.

Clinicians seem to sometimes apply malingering detection methods to conditions that have been minimally studied without sufficient concern about the risky nature of such undertakings. One of the authors was involved in a case in which effort measures were administered to a non-English-speaking group of children and adolescents with questionable exposure to a minimally studied agent. A number of these individuals had limited education, and lived in a war torn, impoverished region of the world that subjected them to an array of risk factors. How could one know what is and is not expectable under such conditions, or what represents sufficient versus insufficient effort (although this did not stop the psychologists who evaluated them from opining about their level of effort and functioning)?

Clearly, certain methods are likely to generalize widely (e.g., scores well below chance are likely to mean the same thing across conditions), but the generalization of other methods and detection strategies is not easily predicted and may have been subjected to minimal or no research. Validity is of course a specific quality and not a global one, and simply because a malingering method works well for a 30-year-old White male with a possible mild head injury does not mean the same will apply for an elderly member of a minority group who appears to have had substantial exposure to a toxin that has been the subject of very few neuropsychological studies. There is often nothing more helpful to malingering detection than increasing our knowledge about neuropsychological disorders and techniques for measuring them. Surely it is much easier to know what is unexpected when one knows a good deal about what to expect.

Absence of Hard Evidence

It is simple to determine if a brain injury is present when an MRI shows unequivocal evidence of damage. Such evidence may fall short of resolving other issues (e.g., the magnitude of functional change), but it certainly can help. Without entering into a conceptual morass here, most determinations by most neuropsychologists in most forensic evaluations go well beyond simple and almost fully objective determinations. Sources of information (e.g., self-report), test performances, clinical observation, cooperation with evaluative procedures, and often interpretive methods (in particular those relying heavily on clinical judgment) all contain subjective elements, and often sizeable ones. In general and all else being equal, the greater the level of subjectivity and inference involved, the harder the decision task.

Cultural Diversity

In one case a neuropsychologist evaluated a male refugee from a remote region of Africa who had applied for political asylum. Complicating this matter was his confessed killing of two individuals, which he claimed was an act of self-defense, something that could easily have been true or false and which could not be decided by the available information. The evaluation was undertaken to appraise this individual's cognitive functioning and psychological status. On one well-known measure, he performed far below the cutoff for malingering, but not below chance level. The neuropsychologist, claiming extensive knowledge of refugee populations, interpreted the outcome as unremarkable and, if anything, indicative of good cooperation. Perhaps the neuropsychologist was correct in countervailing the usual interpretation, but perhaps she was not. Given what was at stake—the likely death of this examinee if he was not granted asylum but returned to his country of origin, versus the possible death of others if he was granted asylum mistakenly—one would like to have a refined body of scientific knowledge available to help guide decision making. Not only was a body of applicable literature lacking, it was difficult to locate even a single peer-reviewed publication directly on topic.

Given changes in the sociodemographics of the United States and litigants seen for neuropsychological evaluation, as well as the substantial international growth of neuropsychology, there is a pressing need for malingering research that addresses the potential impact of ethnicity, race, culture, and a range of other sociodemographic factors. Growing recognition and investigation of the impact that sociodemographic characteristics can have on neuropsychological assessment and test performance has been an important step forward in the field (e.g., Ardila, 2005; Boone, Victor, Wen, Razani, & Ponton, 2007; Byrd, Miller, Reilly, Weber, Wall, & Heaton, 2006; Crowe, Clay, Sawyer, Crowther, & Allman, 2008; Manly & Jacobs, 2002; Razani, Burciaga, Madore, & Wong, 2007), although there is still a great deal of catching up to do. Moreover, in addition to racial and ethnic status, there are additional differentiators and factors that warrant close attention in neuropsychological assessment and the assessment of effort and malingering, such as level of acculturation, language, quality and type of educational experiences, and disability (e.g., hearing/speech/vision) (Brini et al., 2020; Llorente et al., 2017; Reesman et al., 2014; Tan, Burgess, & Green, 2020).

Research directly examining relationships between such sociocultural factors and malingering remains limited, leaving large scientific gaps, and falls far short of our knowledge base pertaining to "mainstream" groups in the United States. Given the frequency with which litigants come from diverse groups and backgrounds, limits in scientific knowledge place practitioners at a considerable disadvantage. Hence, as Bridges and Ahern (2016) state, "There is an urgent need to devote time and attention to more fully exploring racial and ethnic differences across a variety of malingering assessment methods" (p. 454). We do not want to be in a position of using and then proving, which unfortunately is too often the case, as opposed to first proving and then using in the courtroom.

Nijdam-Jones and Rosenfeld's (2017) review of tests and methods used to assess effort among linguistically, ethnically, and culturally diverse samples yielded disconcerting results that speak to these scientific needs. Their review found that "[b]etween two and four studies appeared annually from 2002 through 2008 ($k = 20$), with only a negligible increase to an average of just over four studies per year ($k = 25$) from 2010 through 2015" (p. 1329). Comparing this limited volume of research to the thousands of studies conducted on the assessment of effort and malingering during the same time period with mainstream groups does not seem to reflect positively on our commitment to action that begins to redress gaps in knowledge about diversity issues in this area, in contrast to the greater relative progress seen in multicultural work in other areas of neuropsychology and psychology in general.

If there are many areas of malingering detection that require additional research to further refine knowledge or that remain largely unresolved even after dozens or more studies have been published, what should we assume about the state of knowledge when we may have trouble locating more than an isolated study or two, or cannot find any studies at all, on a particular aspect of malingering detection? Although the relative paucity of research on malingering assessment with diverse groups is a major concern, it also represents an incredible opportunity for productive contribution given the importance of the topic, population trends, and psychologists' and neuropsychologists' impressive record of accomplishment in malingering research.

If there were strong reasons to believe that many or most sociocultural and demographic factors had minimal influence on our methods for evaluating effort, our current scientific limits might not be of such great concern. However, small or negligible impacts, especially across the board, seem rather unlikely, despite some research that, at first glance, might appear to provide some reassuring outcomes (see Bridges & Ahern, 2016). Before addressing some of this research, simple armchair analysis (which we are often reduced to given the state of scientific knowledge) and research on multicultural factors in other areas of neuropsychology and psychology suggest we may well find significant limits in generalization to diverse groups for a number of reasons. Common strategies for malingering detection look for performance well below expectation, performance below chance levels, or performance that deviates from expected or typical patterns (for instance, global deficits following a very specific and circumscribed brain insult, unexpected failures on easy items in contrast to success on considerably harder items, or lack of a negative performance slope in relation to item difficulty). Given more general background knowledge about the impact of multicultural factors in neuropsychology and psychology, there are good reasons to believe that all of these basic approaches to malingering appraisal will be influenced by sociocultural and sociodemographic factors, although in different ways.

Starting with strategies comparing expected and obtained performance levels, it is immediately concerning that numerous studies of ethnic, racial, or linguistic minorities reveal differences across many neuropsychological tests, with minorities generally scoring lower than Whites. (This does not mean we agree with attributions that are sometimes drawn about the bases for differences.[5]) For instance, African Americans tend to score approximately one standard deviation lower on intelligence tests than Whites (Neisser et al., 1996). Similarly, Hispanics, particularly those who are recent immigrants or are less acculturated to the United States rather than second- or third-generation immigrants, tend to score lower on tests of verbal abilities than do Whites. Thus, for example, if a study with the dominant culture suggests that in cases of mild head injury, performance more than two standard deviations below the mean on certain measures raises a fairly strong likelihood of malingering, minority examinees may need to perform only one standard deviation below their mean to meet that criterion. Performance one standard deviation below the mean occurs eight times more often than performance two standard deviations below the mean (approximately 16% of the time versus 2% of the time, assuming a bell curve), and thus the rate of false-positive identification is likely to increase considerably.

Despite these and other concerns, the limited research to date on malingering detection and ethnic or racial status has usually, but not uniformly, yielded comparable outcomes across groups. (Whether comparable outcomes reflect true equivalence or something else will be taken up shortly.) For example, Martin et al. (2019) found that recommended cutoffs for the Test of Memory Malingering (TOMM) also yielded high specificity rates across most groups whose primary language was not English, including individuals from various countries (e.g., Germany, Spain, Argentina, Chile, Peru, and the Netherlands). However, Nijdam-Jones, Rivera, Rosenfeld, and Arango-Lasprilla (2019) found that level of literacy had a sizeable impact on TOMM performance, to the extent that a considerable percentage of normal individuals obtained scores below suggested cutoff points for identifying deficient effort.

Dean et al. (2008) found no significant differences between African American and Hispanic patients on the MMPI-2 Fake Bad Scale, although they excluded all potential subjects involved in legal proceedings. Tsushima and Tsushima (2009) also uncovered no significant differences between Asian and White claimants on various MMPI-2 indicators of response set, such as F and the Fake Bad Scale. All individuals in this study were pursuing compensation claims.

Vilar-Lopez et al. (2007) investigated three symptom validity tests in Spain using three groups of participants: patients with post-concussion syndrome not involved in litigation, patients with post-concussion syndrome involved in litigation, and university students instructed to fake injury. For all three effort tests, the student group scored significantly lower (i.e., more of them performed in the malingering range) than the two patient groups. No significant differences in scores were obtained between the two patient groups. The authors divided the litigating patients into two

---

[5] Description of the literature demonstrating differences in test performance should not be confused with attribution of cause for these differences. For example, it is perfectly compatible to state that studies show differences in performance between two groups on measures of linguistic proficiency and to also state or argue that those differences appear to be due entirely to acculturation or test bias. Although we believe that unwarranted attributions are sometimes drawn about differences in performance levels, we ask readers not to presume such specific positions on our part.

subgroups: those judged likely to be malingering (patients who failed at least two of the three effort tests) and those judged unlikely to be malingering (those who failed no effort tests). These two subgroups differed significantly on all three measures. Further, the subgroup judged likely to be malingering did not differ significantly from the analog malingering group (the students), and the subgroup judged unlikely to be malingering did not differ significantly from the patients who were not involved in litigation. The authors concluded that the three effort tests they investigated are valid for patients in Spain and that approximately 50% of the patients involved in litigation were malingering (absent, of course, independent confirmation of such).

In contrast, other researchers have found differences in effort tests across ethnic groups. For example, Salazar, Lu, Wen, and Boone (2007) analyzed outpatient records from a neuropsychology clinic at a public hospital in Los Angeles. The authors examined nine malingering indices, some derived from common neuropsychological and cognitive tests and others from specific effort tests. Even when controlling for age and education, Hispanics scored significantly lower than Whites on two of the nine indices. Similarly, African Americans scored significantly lower than Whites on four of the nine indices. The authors also examined cutoff scores. They found that for various measures the levels could be *raised* for Whites without sacrificing good specificity, which they defined as a false-positive rate of 10% or lower. In contrast, some cutoffs needed to be lowered for African Americans, Asians, Hispanics, and those for whom English was not their primary language. The authors concluded that effort tests and indices can have value with ethnic, racial, and linguistic minorities, but that many of these measures may require specific adjustments in standard cutoff scores to achieve adequate specificity. Of particular interest, even when average group performances were similar, the differing score distributions that sometimes occurred still necessitated adjustments in cutoff levels for minority groups to maintain adequate specificity. Such results call into question the conclusions that are often drawn from studies showing no significant group differences between minorities and nonminorities. Salazar et al. noted that the examination of group differences based only on performance averages is insufficient to demonstrate equivalence across ethnic and linguistic groups on effort test performance.

Nijdam-Jones and Rosenfeld's (2017) aforementioned review of cross-cultural research on malingering detection raised a number of methodological concerns, such as reliance on clinical or subjective judgment for determining "known" groups, sample size limitations, and potential problems adapting procedures for different groups. Moreover, the frequency of specific measures examined in the studies under review did not necessarily align with the measures most commonly used in the United States (LaDuke, Barr, Brodale, & Rabin, 2018), e.g., the Structured Inventory of Malingered Symptomatology was examined nearly four times more often than the Minnesota Multiphasic Inventory-2-Restructured Form. Lastly, although obtained specificities for measures were often high or very high, a number of measures yielded concerning outcomes, such as the Dot Counting Test (0.73), Reliable Digit Span (0.75), and the Miller Forensic Assessment of Symptoms Test (0.74). It is also often the case that error rates obtained in studies often seem to underestimate error rates in common applications in practice (see the latter discussion of the extreme group problem). Given such considerations, it would seem highly probable that if one follows certain guides, such as drawing a strong conclusion about poor effort or malingering if an examinee obtains even a few results signaling inadequate effort, then a false-positive error rate of about 25% across a series of effort tests will produce an alarming rate of misdiagnosis. Here, such errors would be misidentifying individuals who are making satisfactory effort as noncooperative or malingering.

Perhaps of even greater concern than strategies that compare performance *levels* to expectation are approaches that emphasize deviation from expected test *patterns*, and especially those that place heavy reliance on impressionistic or clinical judgment. Some formal methods for appraising deviation from expected patterns (e.g., performance curves that comport with item difficulty) are well grounded scientifically, at least for use with members of the mainstream or "dominant" culture (e.g., Frederick, 2003). These formal methods tend to focus on one or a few dimensions rather than complex pattern analysis. In contrast, the common recommendation to perform complex pattern analysis using clinical judgment conflicts with a large body of literature raising powerful concerns about the ability to execute such approaches successfully. Further, hundreds of studies show that simpler methods, and more specifically properly developed statistical decision procedures or actuarial methods, almost always equal or exceed the accuracy of clinical judgment (see "Data Combination" and "Research on Complex Data Integrative Capacities" above). Unfortunately, survey research suggests that many neuropsychologists place greater emphasis on subjective strategies for malingering assessment and pattern analysis than on formal methods with considerably stronger scientific support (see Sharland & Gfeller, 2007).

As we have noted, there are powerful obstacles to *complex* pattern analysis in psychology and neuropsychology. We previously discussed the cognitive limits of decision makers, but there are also a number of major psychometric obstacles. For example, a significant body of evidence suggests that many forms of pattern analysis are unreliable (Watkins, Glutting, & Youngstrom, 2005). There is simply too much error in individual test scores that gets compounded when comparing results across multiple tests, even despite attempts to add redundancy to the procedures, making patterns difficult to discern in even rather straightforward cases.

Problems with complex pattern analysis are compounded when evaluations involve racial, ethnic, and cultural factors. Unless there are no effects from these variables or the effects are equal across tests and subtests, the inevitable result is to alter patterns. To take a simple example, suppose in cases of suspected mild head injury, performance on test A that exceeds performance on test B by more than one standard deviation is a potential indicator of malingering. Assume now that within a certain group, in comparison to members of the dominant culture, individuals average higher performance on test A and lower performance on test B. Hence, using norms for the dominant culture, a large number of individuals who are not malingering may exceed this level of discrepancy across the tests.

Although diminished performance is often the focus of attention when cultural differences are described, such alterations are usually not constant across tests (see

Bridges & Ahern, 2016; Faust et al., 2011; Hambleton, Merenda, & Spielberger, 2005; Heaton, Ryan, & Grant, 2009; Rosselli, & Ardila, 2003). For some tests the disadvantages may be relatively large, for others minimal or absent, and for still other tests members of a certain cultural group may outperform the members of the dominant culture. It is probably evident that these unequal influences can grossly distort or alter patterns. Furthermore, in many instances, there is little or no research on the impact of culture on some or most of the tests that are being administered, and thus any such influences are unknown, or common beliefs lack sufficient scientific foundations. For example, many psychologists believe, and proceed as if, cultural influences can be reduced or minimized by using nonverbal tests. However, this assumption is often counterfactual: equal or greater influences may be observed on such tests, and so-called nonverbal tests also often contain innate linguistic demands (Ardila, 2007; Hambleton et al., 2005; Heaton, Ryan, & Grant, 2009; Nabors, Evans, & Strickland, 2000; Rosselli & Ardila, 2003). More generally, attempts to identify malingering that depend on complex pattern analysis in members of nondominant cultural or ethnic groups may fall short of even educated guesses, and regrettably reflect the readiness of some experts to proceed almost no matter how deficient their scientific bases may be, and even in the face of considerable evidence contradicting their assumptions.

An additional or supplemental approach to malingering detection emphasizes diagnostic criteria or guidelines, which often have equivocal supportive evidence in the first place but may become even more questionable when applied to minority groups. Sbordone, Strickland, and Purish (2000) addressed criteria for malingering detection that have appeared across multiple editions of the *Diagnostic and Statistical Manual* (up to and including the current edition, *DSM-5*, American Psychiatric Association, 2013). The criteria include: (a) medicolegal context; (b) antisocial personality disorder; (c) marked discrepancy between claimed stress or disability and objective findings; and (d) lack of cooperation with evaluation and treatment. Each of these has been found to be more prevalent in ethnic and racial minorities than in Whites. Ethnic minorities are overrepresented in medicolegal settings, particularly the criminal context (Sbordone et al., 2000). Fewer educational opportunities and lower academic achievement also translate into a greater representation of ethnic and racial minorities in blue-collar jobs or manual labor—precisely the sorts of jobs that are more likely to result in physical injury and subsequent litigation than are white-collar or office/clerical jobs.

A diagnosis of antisocial personality disorder is sometimes thought to relate to malingering because people with this diagnosis have fewer qualms about lying or cheating to achieve personal gains. However, Sbordone et al. pointed out that the *DSM* criteria for diagnosing antisocial personality disorder focus on behavioral rather than characterological traits, such as repeatedly engaging in illegal or aggressive activities or failure to maintain a job or fulfill financial obligations (a point that applies similarly to the updated version of the DSM, or DSM-5). Such behaviors can also be educed by growing up in an impoverished environment in which few options for employment, financial affluence, or prosocial behavior are present. Unfortunately, poverty disproportionately affects ethnic and racial minorities

(Kaiser Family Foundation, 2011). Therefore, behaviors used to identify antisocial disorder may occur more often in ethnic or racial minorities due to more trying life circumstances rather than a desire to manipulate or con others, a lack of empathy, or an underdeveloped conscience.

Sbordone et al. (2000) noted that the discrepancy between subjective impairment and objective findings is a hallmark of many psychiatric disorders, not only of malingering. The authors argued that minorities and the poor are overrepresented in various psychiatric categories, and thus using this criterion as a marker of malingering could be ill-founded. They further observed that inadequate compliance with evaluation and treatment also might prove problematic as an indicator of malingering among ethnic or racial minorities. Ample research documents the underutilization of health and mental health services among minorities—they are less likely to seek services, more likely to drop out early from recommended treatments, and more likely to be considered noncompliant with treatment than are Whites (Nelson, 2002; Satcher, 2001). The primary reasons for such noncompliance do not appear to be malingering, but rather economic and cultural barriers, such as inadequate health insurance coverage; low availability of trusted, culturally competent healthcare providers; transportation barriers; and linguistic barriers.

Thus, for each one of the four criteria, ethnic and racial minorities may be overrepresented due to cultural and financial factors rather than feigning disability, illness, or attempting to manipulate others for personal gain. Given these concerns, Sbordone et al. (2000) concluded that falsely labeling someone as a malingerer is significantly more likely to occur for ethnic minority examinees.

Rogers (1990a, 1990b) has long criticized these four criteria, including their application to ethnic majority members, and instead suggested that certain circumstances may create motivation to exaggerate or malinger. Specifically, Rogers suggested that adversarial circumstances, in which individuals believe they have much to lose by being fully forthcoming, and where alternative means of achieving a goal are not perceived as viable or effective, increase the likelihood of malingering. When one considers life experiences, it seems likely that the adversarial nature of legal proceedings may impact minority examinees disproportionately. For instance, poverty and discrimination (perceived or actual) create precisely the sort of adversarial conditions in which a minority examinee might be powerfully tempted to exaggerate in order to diminish the perceived risk of victimization. Is it truly fair to equate an attempt to overreport in order to be treated *fairly* when one may have repeatedly experienced discrimination and has come to expect its occurrence with overreporting in order to get more than one deserves? Trials, at their core, are morality plays.

Salazar et al. (2007) argued that the motives underlying malingering, such as monetary gain, avoidance of criminal prosecution or work, and opportunities to improve life circumstances, are "universal temptations" (p. 405). However, researchers investigating malingering in minority groups often seem to assume that frequencies are comparable in minority and majority group members. A typical study of malingering detection compares performance levels or failure rates on effort tests in minority and nonminority groups and, if no significant differences are found, concludes that the test is valid for minority populations. The problem with such reasoning is its tautological nature: It takes as a given a premise that has not really been tested, that is, that malingering rates are constant across the groups. For example, if the rate is lower among minority groups, obtaining comparable outcomes on measures may reflect a high frequency of false-positive error, or if the rate is lower the converse may apply (i.e., false-negative rates may be elevated). Until adequate base rate information on malingering is obtained, such interpretations of study outcomes lack the needed foundations. So much research in so many areas shows ethnic or racial differences, it is sensible to expect that such differences may well appear across malingering detection methods, until or unless proven otherwise.

We commend the research being done in the area of malingering detection and ethnicity, but also realize it is still generally in an early stage and that much work lies ahead both conceptually and methodologically. For instance, studies have thus far tended to lump together all members of a particular group (e.g., using categories such as "Asians" or "Hispanics") and ignored within-group differences. In many cases, differences within groups, especially when groups are identified broadly or with a degree of arbitrariness, can equal or exceed differences across groups. For example, who necessarily has more in common: a Spanish-speaking CEO in a major corporation in Barcelona and an English-speaking CEO in a major corporation in New York, or that same Spanish-speaking CEO and a Spanish-speaking Central American living in an impoverished and extremely remote village, with no formal education or access to social media?

Even when studies demonstrate no differences in group means, more nuanced analyses of test sensitivity suggest that cutoff scores on malingering tests should be adjusted for different minority groups. It is plausible to conjecture that generalization will differ across measures, detection strategies, and cultural and language differences. For example, finding that a method generalizes reasonably well to highly acculturated individuals provides minimal assurance the same will hold with other groups. Will a method that depends on the analysis of discrepancies across four tests derived from research with mainstream Americans work similarly when used, for example, with an adolescent from Somalia who lived in a refugee camp for 2 years before immigrating to the United States 6 months previously? Patterns of test performance can shift dramatically under altered conditions, so how favorable are the odds that a detection method that depends on deviation from expected highs and lows will apply unaltered?

Major variables that may better account for minority group differences, such as poverty, educational attainment, and acculturation, remain understudied. Finally, the unstated assumption that malingering rates are the same in minorities as nonminorities may not be tenable and, in any case, often cannot be tested sufficiently at present given limitations in the state of knowledge. Situations many minority examinees face, such as mistrusting the legal or medical system, attempting to avoid being labeled, fighting potential discrimination and stigma, or harboring concerns that one's difficulties will not be understood by another, all create circumstances in which exaggeration or dissimulation seem more likely to occur. Both the National Academy of Neuropsychology's (NAN's) position paper on malingering detection

(Bush et al., 2005) and the American Academy of Clinical Neuropsychology's consensus statement (Heilbronner et al., 2009) raise concerns about cultural influences on the outcome of malingering tests. As stated in the NAN paper, "Simply because a SVT [symptom validity test] has been validated in the majority culture does not mean that the test is equally valid with individuals from a minority culture" (p. 425).

Subtlety of Presentation/Relevant Differentials

Close calls and subtle conditions (but those that can still exercise substantial impact on personal, social, or occupational functioning) usually create greater difficulties than extreme cases. As a parallel and obvious example, it is much easier to identify advanced Alzheimer's disease than early cases. Similarly, it is much easier to separate individuals with severe brain injuries from normal individuals than to differentiate individuals with mild brain injuries from those who may have somewhat low functional baselines but are not injured. Much malingering research is compromised by the use of subjects and presentations that are rather extreme and distinct from the closer calls that often arise in contested legal cases. The latter instances often involve individuals for whom there are fairly strong reasons to suspect malingering, some of whom are malingering and some of whom are not, and some of whom are injured and some of whom are not. As we now turn our attention to research needs, these closer calls and the need to simultaneously address both malingering and injury will come to the forefront of our discussion.

5   Research Factors and Pressing Needs

The third section of Table 1 lists additional factors that contribute to false-negative and false-positive errors and sets forth what we believe to be high priorities for continued or concentrated research efforts. We will cover these entries in order, some of which are broadly recognized, but others that have been less completely or minimally described.

5.1   Mixed Presentations: *Injured* and *Malingering*

A litigant should not have to qualify for sainthood to be compensated fairly for genuine injury. Litigants do not find themselves in a legal system that approaches moral and functional perfection, in which virtually all experts perform nearly flawless evaluations and proceed with unwavering objectivity and fairness, thereby minimizing concerns that symptom complaints or test performances reflecting true injury will not be given their just due. Despite what can be the impressive moral character of litigants, excellent mechanisms for resolving legal disputes, and proficient experts who strive for fairness, we are fallible individuals in fallible systems that sometimes misstep and diverge far from the ideal. Given these realities, we require tolerance of and adjustment for the human condition to maximize just outcomes.

This is not to suggest that a person should be compensated for a feigned injury. Furthermore, in cases of genuine injury, a good argument can be made for subtracting something from the level of compensation when elements of exaggeration are present. Such elements can have deleterious impact on the legal system and society and, among other things, we wish to deter these sorts of behaviors. However, there are compelling reasons to argue for reasonable proportionality between the presence, extent, and type of falsification and the adverse consequences that ought to result. For example, a hardened criminal who falsely accuses a therapist of depraved behavior simply to receive a financial payoff can hardly be grouped with someone who has suffered a severe injury and embellishes just a little when evaluated by a defense expert who has a well-deserved reputation for underestimating loss. It is for these and other reasons that identifying exaggeration or falsification, in and of itself, may fall well short of providing adequate information for appraising a litigant, and why neuropsychologists need to be concerned about joint presentations, especially the co-occurrence of malingering and injury.

If we do not accept the extreme position that *any* degree of falsification should disqualify individuals from *all* compensation, then enhancing knowledge of joint presentations may be recognized as something that could be of great practical value and should be given high research priority. It is precisely because injury status and malingering have partial independence from one another that determining whether someone is malingering often will not resolve questions about the presence or extent of injury. Nevertheless, laypersons may tend to see the categories as mutually exclusive or mostly so (and sometimes are inappropriately encouraged to do so by experts), which is one reason research on mixed presentations seems so important. The contribution of forensic experts to just outcomes is proportionate to the degree their knowledge exceeds the ken of laypersons on issues critical to legal disputes, and hence advances in research knowledge and clinical practice in this area could provide major benefits.

We wish to be quite clear that we are not endorsing or excusing embellishment or falsification, but we also think it is puritanical, categorically unwise, counterproductive, and often simply unfair to lump all such acts together. Rather, many such actions fall within the range of normal human failings and may be elicited, as Rogers (1990a, 1990b) noted decades earlier, by contextual factors. To illustrate, take an item on the MMPI-2 (Butcher, Graham, Ben-Porath, Tellegen, Dahlstrom, & Kaemmer, 2001) which asks whether one believes that most people will lie to avoid problems. Among contemporary samples of patient and nonpatient groups, between 50% and 60% of individuals responded affirmatively. For an item asking whether the respondent has pretended to be ill to avoid some responsibility, between 59% and 68% of the groups answered affirmatively. Should a neuropsychologist take a rigid stance about such matters, we suggest that he or she might be administered the "test" we have designed and present in Table 4. The first two items are modeled after

Table 4 The malingering/credibility test for experts

Items
I have never told people I was sick in order to avoid some activity I didn't care to do. (Faking illness for self-gain.)
I would never avoid paying every last cent in taxes I legitimately owe even if I were positive I would get away with it. (Stealing, avoidance of social responsibility.)
I have never taken something like a bar of soap, a small bottle of shampoo, a towel, or a hanger from any hotel room any time in my life. (Stealing.)
I have never exaggerated any of my accomplishments or qualities, e.g., my grades, how well I handled some situation, how considerate I was of others, my work performance, etc. (Exaggerating positive qualities; covering up negative qualities.)
If I were stopped going well over the speed limit and a police officer admitted the radar gun was broken, I would still report my speed to the best of my ability. (Trying to get around the law.)
If a bank executive was interviewing me for a loan I really wanted, I would never say anything good about the bank if I had even the slightest reservations. (Lying for monetary gain.)
When my parents asked me what I was going to do when I said I was going out, I told them the complete truth every time. (Lying to others; manipulating others.)
When people ask me about my history, I divulge everything, no matter how bad or embarrassing it might be. (Providing a misleading history; not admitting to personal shortcomings.)
On first dates, I never tried to create an impression that was even a little more positive than was truly accurate. (Manipulating others for personal gain.)
When I was interviewed for graduate school, I was completely frank in responding to all interview questions and made no effort to emphasize my strengths and downplay my weaknesses. (Misleading others for self-gain.)
Interpretive guide
Given the low sensitivity of the test, a negative answer to any item raises a strong suspicion of falsification (simulation) and doubt about all results. Conversely, any positive response demonstrates an unwillingness to admit to personal shortcomings (dissimulation). If manipulation of results is found, the expert is subject to penalty, such as forfeiture of all expert fees earned over the last 5 years.

questions from the MMPI-2. Table 4 is intended to bring home the point that not all forms of impression management are equivalent or a basis for denying all compensation for true injury. It might be argued that the entries in Table 4 are absurd or pedestrian, which is exactly as intended.

Especially considering our adversarial system in which the attorney is expected to put on the best case possible, plaintiffs who do not exhibit an iota of impression management, overstatement, or exaggeration (i.e., present nothing but injury with a complete absence of spin) are almost certainly the exception, and in many other cases individuals who are clearly exaggerating or falsifying have also suffered some degree of injury. The great majority of cases likely falls between the extremes and involves some combination of injury and impression management or exaggeration. The frequency of such mixed cases has profound implications for mental health professionals involved in legal cases and for researchers. These cases create assessment challenges and critical scientific needs that have been grossly understudied. The fundamental scientific agenda is to devise ways to separate out, to the extent possible, legitimate injury attributable to the event in question from pseudo-injury or false elements, and thereby deliver useable and effective tools for clinicians. The fundamental task and moral agenda of the trier of fact is to try to sort out these legitimate and nonlegitimate elements, and to then apply what has been discerned to deciding liability and damage issues. For the trier of fact, undertaking both factual and moral determinations is congruent with assigned roles because, after all, the normative justification for the legal system is fair dispute resolution.

Whether or not technically appropriate, the manner in which a judge or juror sorts through the litigant's credibility in the area of damages may have a decisive effect on all major elements of the case, including liability. The spillover to liability issues may occur because such determinations often depend largely on the plaintiff's description given the absence or ambiguity of corroborating evidence. For example, the plaintiff may state that she slipped on a patch of ice and not simply over her own two feet, or that some power tool that was supposed to shut off under certain circumstances failed to do so. In the area of damages, many self-reports or symptom complaints (e.g., trouble sleeping) cannot be independently verified. Thus, in general, a plaintiff whose credibility is viewed as questionable or poor may be compensated well below fair value because subjective complaints that cannot be verified objectively are not believed, or may not be compensated at all, no matter the merits of the case and the occurrence of genuine injury.

These matters should concern experts because it may be their results and testimony that help to sway jurors. Obviously, valid conclusions can foster just resolution of cases and errors can move outcomes in the wrong direction. More so, by identifying and explaining mixed presentations and subtler distinctions or combinations, experts may be able to correct overly polarized views of credibility that conceptualize the matter as all or none or that tend to place credibility and injury in opposition to one another. Of course, if the field fails to develop the needed scientific knowledge on mixed presentation or experts adopt overly narrow views of such matters themselves, what is being offered in this domain may do little to enhance the average layperson's understanding. It is because mixed presentations likely occur with regularity, judgments of credibility have such a powerful impact on cases, misconceptualization in this area might be common, and there is so little direct scientific research on the topic that we consider it a pressing research need. For example, as we will discuss, accurate determinations of base rates and the proficiency of detection methods will likely depend heavily on accounting for mixed presentations, and what we do find may show that certain current beliefs are often off by a wide margin.

Variations in Conjoint Presentations

We ask readers to look back at Figs. 2 and 3. Figure 2 subdivides groups along a series of dimensions, with the third line representing litigants who undergo neuropsychological evaluation. Of those individuals, some will have brain injury and some will not, and within each of those two subgroups, some will malinger or exaggerate and some will not. As carried over into Fig. 3, the possible combinations of these two conditions or dimensions result in four admittedly simplified categories: not injured and not malingering (I−/M−), not injured and malingering (I−/M+), injured and not malingering (I+/M−), and both injured and malingering (M+/I+). Although of secondary importance for the moment, the cases within each category can be subdivided into those that can be identified definitively or nearly definitively (D/ND) and those that are more difficult to identify or are more ambiguous (AMB). Given the particular difficulty they present, the AMB cases are of greater applied research interest than cases we are already able to identify accurately (the latter of which often is a result of advances researchers have achieved).

The lower section of Fig. 3 sets forth the four possible combinations of accurate and inaccurate decisions for each category and its associated standing on the dual dimensions of injury and malingering. For example, for individuals who are neither malingering nor injured, judgments about both dimensions may be correct (Acc/Acc), they may both be incorrect (Inacc/Inacc), or judgments about either injury or malingering may be incorrect. For those less familiar with the terminology adopted in Fig. 3, VN (valid negative) represents an accurate judgment that a condition is absent, VP (valid positive) an accurate judgment that a condition is present, FN (false negative) an inaccurate judgment that a condition is absent, and FP (false positive) an inaccurate judgment that a condition is present. Unlike simple dichotomous choices in which random selection yields a 50% accuracy rate, given the four possibilities, chance level is only 25% (and the corresponding error rate 75%). Thus, the need for help in decision making is magnified when dual identifications are at issue.

Arguably, some types of errors may be more harmful than others, partly depending on the setting or context of decision making. For example, in a criminal context, an individual who does not have a condition that may compromise judgment or impulse control and who is not malingering, and yet is mistakenly identified as a falsifier, may be unjustly denied release. In a clinical context, this error may not cause nearly as much harm to someone who is not injured as it would to a person who is injured and is falsely identified as a malingerer.

Additionally, judgments on one dimension may interact with judgments about the other dimension and do so in an unorthodox manner. In Fig. 3, some combinations of the injury/malingering categories and decision accuracy status are bounded by different shapes, each of which identifies different possible interactions. Some errors on one dimension increase the probability that judgments about the other dimension will also be *incorrect*, but other errors increase the probability that judgments about the other dimension will be *correct*. For some combinations, *correct* judgments about the first dimension increase the probability that judgments about the other dimension will be *incorrect*. At others times, the accuracy of a decision on either of the two dimensions is unlikely to affect accuracy on the other dimension.

For example, take the third column, I+/M−, and the entry within it enclosed by a rectangle, FN/FP. This tells us it is quite possible that if one makes a false-negative error when appraising injury, the risk of a false-positive error when appraising malingering is elevated. In this case, abnormal test results are not believed to be associated with true injury or perhaps do not seem to fit with expectations for head injury, and hence the odds of falsely identifying them as a product of malingering are likely to increase. Here, error leads to more error. In contrast, look at the first column, I−/M−, and the entry enclosed by an oval, FP/VN. It is quite possible that if one makes a false-positive error in identifying injury, there is an increased likelihood that the absence of malingering will be identified correctly. Here, the first error may decrease the frequency with which the second type of error is made. Ironically, even correct judgments about one dimension may increase the chances of error on the other dimension. For example, consider the fourth column, I+/M+, and the entry labeled VP/FN (in a hexagon). Here, the correct identification of injury may lead to more frequent false-negative errors when appraising malingering. Thus, we may have incorrect judgments compounding or counteracting other potential errors, or even correct judgments on one dimension leading to greater error rates on the other dimension. Although other and more complex forms of interrelationships between correct and incorrect judgments may well occur, to our knowledge not even such rudimentary and sometimes paradoxical relationships have been subjected to needed investigation. It is additionally disconcerting to think that these same sorts of interactions between correct and incorrect judgments may be passed along to jurors or reinforce their own misconceptions. Consequently, rather than helping to sort through potential confusion, experts may at times compound misunderstandings. It will take high-quality science to begin sorting through these complexities.

Conjoint Presentations: Limits in Knowledge and Potential Consequences

We seem to know remarkably little about joint presentations, including such basic matters as their relative frequency, the resultant distributions of scores on standard tests and tests designed specifically to detect malingering, and the accuracy with which they are identified. Differences in hypothetical expected test results for our four joint injury/malingering presentations are illustrated in Fig. 5. This example assumes a mild traumatic brain injury (mTBI) is at issue. For purposes of simplification, the figure illustrates expected standing on only a single test of ability, one that uses a forced-choice procedure. Certainly things become much more complex when multiple assessment tools are used and a much larger data base has been gathered, and the differential may include a variety of plausible possibilities alone or in combination, such as head injury plus history of alcohol abuse plus history of mood disorder. In Fig. 5, higher scores, or scores representing better performance, are represented to the left and lower scores to the right. As illustrated, scores for each group may extend over all or part of the normal range, the abnormal range, or a range that falls below chance performance. The shaded areas represent ranges for which determinations of true status are likely to be most difficult for each I/M presentation.

The I−/M− group generally obtains normal scores although, as is common on many tests, a relatively small subset falls in the abnormal range. That small subset risks being misdiagnosed as either injured or malingering.

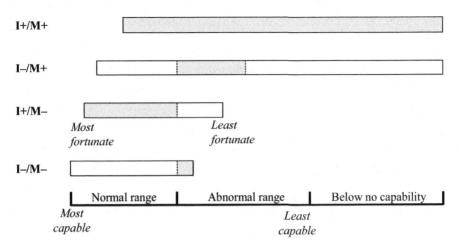

Fig. 5 Performance on a quantitative indicator of mild brain injury showing areas of concern (shaded) for identifying Injured/Malingering subgroups

Assuming the capacity being evaluated is often affected in a subset of individuals with mTBI who do not make good recoveries, the I+/M− group obtains lower scores than the normal group, a greater frequency of abnormal results, and a broader range of scores. There will be considerable overlap across the groups, and error is most likely to occur when a normal individual performs in the abnormal range or an injured individual performs in the normal range. We understand that deficits following mild head injury can be selective. However, for purposes of this example it should be assumed that some members of the head-injured group have suffered chronic loss in functioning, and for those individuals a normal score represents a false-negative finding when considered relative to overall status. (Alternatively, one could assume this is a cumulative index comprised of tests of demonstrated sensitivity to the effects of head injury, all of which use a forced-choice format. However, such details do not change the fundamental situation and are unimportant for the illustrative intent of Fig. 5.)

The I−/M+ group may well demonstrate a very wide range of performance, with some individuals, perhaps those who are high functioning and rather selective when feigning deficit, performing somewhat below their baseline but still well within normal limits. The shaded area of the bar for this group falls at a level sufficiently deviant to suggest abnormality but not so extreme as to suggest, or strongly suggest, malingering.

Finally, the I+/M+ group, having both true injury and deliberately not performing up to their capability, almost must obtain scores that on average fall at a lower level than the I+/M− group. Additionally, they are likely to show a very wide distribution of scores. However, unlike the other three groups, with somewhat narrow bands within which determinations may cause the greatest difficulty, for the I+/M+ group the entire range of performance is of concern. This is because even a relatively strong performance does not rule out a drop from baseline functioning, and even the poorest score does not rule out a degree of true injury. In fact, it is wrong to conclude either that there is no true injury or that depressed scores are due to malingering. Additionally, recognizing that some component of diminished performance may be or clearly is due to inadequate effort is not necessarily that helpful, and making finer discriminations is highly desirable. For example, if in one case we are dealing with 90% malingering and 10% true injury, we probably do not want to group it with another case in which we are dealing with 90% injury and 10% exaggeration, particularly if, in the latter case, even subtle or minor deficits have created major alterations in functioning (e.g., an airline pilot who cannot return to work).

It is natural to ask what scientific knowledge base could differentiate between malingering *or* injured versus malingering *and* injured and, in the case of joint presentations, assist in appraising proportionality. As a profession, we might throw up our hands and say it is not possible. However, there are certainly instances in other domains in which level of over- or underreporting is measured and the attempt is made, at least if neither is too extreme, to apply corrective measures or adjustments (e.g., the MMPI-2 K scale). More so, why give up on the challenge before we have really started, especially given the serious implications of incomplete knowledge in this area. Until we know the base rates for mixed presentations and our accuracy in identifying them, estimates that have otherwise been provided for malingering and the accuracy of measures are like solving for X with not one but two elements missing—it cannot be done. The consequence is to render assertions about how well we do in this domain, the degree of accuracy that measures achieve, or attempts to incorporate base rates into decision procedures crude guesses or worse.

Let us illustrate the basis for these concerns. Suppose an author claims that the base rate for malingering is 25% in a forensic population and that one or another malingering measure is accurate in 70% of cases. Aside from previously raised concerns about the accuracy of such estimates and the overriding need to determine base rates for appropriate subgroups, such figures are likely to disregard mixed presentations. First, we do not know what proportion of this 25% also have nontrivial injuries. Second, given the propensity to treat malingering as merely a present/absent phenomenon and to set high thresholds for identifying its presence, we also do not know what percentage of individuals considered nonmalingerers (the remaining 75%) also show mixed features. Third, assuming interest in identifying mixed presentations, we have virtually no evidence on this matter either relating to the base rates or the accuracy of identification. If both malingering and injury status are highly relevant concerns, as we have argued they often are, it is not clear just how far the available information gets us, especially when one starts to explore the range of possible subgroup frequencies.

To further clarify the possible impact of mixed presentations and their occurrence rates, assume in some setting the frequency of malingering is 50%. Assume further that within this group, those that are malingering only and are *not* also injured (M+/I−) can be identified with 80% accuracy. In contrast, those that are malingering *and* are injured (M+/I+) are rarely identified correctly, with accuracy rates falling only at 10%. Given these assumptions, it is possible to examine what occurs as the base rate for the M+/I+ group shifts. (We sometimes alter the order in which malingering and injury status are listed solely for expository purposes, but this change is not meant to convey any substantive difference.)

Suppose that within the overall group of malingerers, 90% are M+/I− cases (are not also injured) and 10% are M+/I+ cases (are also injured). Projecting across 100 cases, the 90 M+/I− cases are identified with 80% accuracy, resulting in 90 × .80, or 72 correct identifications; and the 10 M+/I+ cases are identified with 10% accuracy, resulting in 10 × .10, or 1 additional correct identification. The combined result is 72 + 1 = 73 correct identifications, or a 73% accuracy rate. In comparison to the 80% accuracy rate for identifying malingering alone, the combined rate of 73% is not quite as good but still well above chance level. However, what if 40% of the overall group of malingerers are M+/I+ cases, or also have significant injuries? Under such circumstances, 80% of the 60 M+/I− are classified accurately, resulting in 48 correct identifications, but only 10% of the 40 I+/M+ cases are classified accurately, resulting in 4 correct identifications. The combined total is 52 correct identifications, or a 52% accuracy rate, which is just about at chance level.

To the extent the base rate for M+/I+ cases increases, the situation only deteriorates further. Suppose the overall group is comprised of 80% M+/I+ cases. Given this base rate, 16 of the M+/I− cases are classified correctly (20 cases × .80) and 8 of the M+/I+ cases (80 cases × .10), yielding an abysmal overall accuracy rate of 24%. To determine which, if any, of such hypothetical figures holds, one must know such things as the base rate for the M+/I+ group in the setting of interest, and yet our knowledge about such matters is sorely deficient. Although purely anecdotal, one of the authors has asked various plaintiff and defense lawyers what they believe is the most common presentation in personal injury cases. Every one responded that it was probably the I+/M+ group, or that among those who are truly injured, most show some degree of embellishment or falsification given the nature of the adversarial system.

More generally, our accuracy rates are a combined product of the base rates for the different joint presentations and how well we identify each subgroup. Suppose, for example, that accuracy in identifying three of the four groups is 80% for each group and that the base rates for the three groups are about equal. In contrast, accuracy in identifying the I+/M+ group is only at chance level. If the base rate for the I+/M+ group is 10%, the combined accuracy rate (for all four subgroups) will be about 75%, well above the level possible by playing the base rates. Specifically, across 100 cases, the other three groups will make up 90 cases and the I+/M+ group 10 cases. If the 90 other cases are identified with 80% accuracy, then .80 × 90 cases will be identified correctly, or 72 cases. If the 10 I+/M+ cases are identified at chance level, which, given four possible choices or groups is 25%, then .25 × 10, or about 2–3 additional cases will be identified correctly. Combining the 72 correct identifications for the other cases and the 2–3 correct identifications for the I+/M+ cases results in 74–75 correct identifications out of 100, or about a 75% accuracy rate. If one plays the base rates, one selects the most frequent outcome. If the other three cases are distributed about equally and hence each occurs about 30% of the time, the accuracy achieved playing the base rates is only 30%.

It is disconcerting to examine what occurs if the base rate for the I+/M+ increases. For example, if the base rate for the I+/M+ group is 25%, the overall accuracy rate for all four groups combined decreases to about 66%; if it is as high as 70%, which may not be outlandish in some situations, overall accuracy declines to about 42%. (These frequencies can be derived by following the same steps set forth above for the 10% base rate.) Obviously, shifting assumptions about relative frequencies and accuracy rates for subgroups changes projections, but the disquieting fact is that we really have little idea what figures might apply. The I+/M+ group may be common and perhaps as or more frequent than any of the other subgroups, and yet it is far and away the least studied. This problem is greatly confounded by research designs that emphasize pure or extreme groups and thereby may inadvertently focus on less frequently occurring and nonrepresentative presentations, consequently distorting and limiting our knowledge base. (Additional serious consequences of what we refer to as the *Extreme Group Problem* will be described below.)

Implications of Conjoint Presentations for Clinical and Research

When pondering possible research and clinical approaches for these joint presentations, it quickly becomes clear that we are entering deep waters. This complexity is evident when one considers how simplified the previous discussion has been, focusing, for example, on single variables for exemplars, emphasizing dichotomous categories versus matters of degree, and not even touching on critical factors arising from distributions as opposed to simple ranges. We will attempt to describe some key issues and leave more detailed discussion for a later planned work.

With two dichotomous possibilities (again simplifying for the moment), one can sometimes go a long way toward decreasing uncertainty or at least resolving pragmatic concerns by making a single correct choice. For example, if one can determine definitively or nearly definitively that someone was not injured, a critical question has been answered and the issue of malingering may become moot. If head injury is ruled out, then whether an individual is malingering might make little difference, and there may be no point in performing testing at all. Suppose the site at which the individual claims to have fallen and sustained a head injury is monitored with a video camera, the tape is available, and it is clear the head was not impacted at all and that a head injury could not have occurred. There is no point in conducting neuropsychological testing to determine if a brain injury resulted from the event because one already knows it is not the case, and if testing yielded an abnormal result there would have to be some other cause. If no testing is conducted, the hypothetical possibility of insufficient effort on testing becomes moot.

Assuming the definitive video is unavailable (which it almost never is), other information will still sometimes allow a near-definitive determination. One seeks information that *maximizes diagnostic validity* and *minimizes susceptibility to manipulation*. For example, although the presence and length of post-traumatic amnesia have considerable diagnostic value, self-report of such is highly susceptible to manipulation. It is no revelation to say that the same individual who might purposely underperform on tests might also provide misleading information about alterations in cognitive functioning at the time of the accident. In contrast, other sources of information (e.g., the observations of trained professionals at the scene who are motivated to reach the correct conclusions, or information about the individual's actions at the time), while subject to error, are almost certainly less likely to be purposely altered to create false impressions. On occasion, rich sources of dependable information are available that allow one to rule out a head injury with a high level of certainty. We understand that error or manipulation can enter into these matters as well, such as when an individual stages an accident and pretends to be unconscious. However, fallibility and lack of utility should not be conflated, nor are all fallible methods equal because some are far more fallible than are others.

At times, other sources of information, even if minimally susceptible to manipulation, may not help much. If, for example, the occurrence of a mild head injury is in question, a normal CT scan will not get us very far, despite what some individuals might still think, as would also be true of a negative EEG when seizure disorder is questioned. No matter how impressive certain technology might appear, when the task is to all but definitively rule out one or the other dichotomous choice, false-negative error rates beyond a very low level are essentially fatal.

Although *ruling out* the injury in question usually resolves major questions, *ruling in* the injury may have surprisingly limited value. Suppose in the case of a small depressed skull fracture, scanning demonstrates a highly localized but unquestionable area of brain damage. This unfortunate occurrence has now been established, but the situation is unlike one in which injury has been ruled out and concerns about malingering often become secondary. Instead, the co-occurrence of malingering can be highly relevant and could even be the major determinant of self-report, test performance, and other manifestations of seeming dysfunction. The potential presence and impact of fabrication remain ambiguous to the extent that evidence about the presence of structural injury, despite perhaps being highly trustworthy, is not sufficiently predictive of functional consequences. In many cases, knowledge of structural alteration does not provide a strong basis for predicting or determining functional consequences, especially if injuries are not extreme or occur in certain brain regions, or if one tries to project over longer time intervals. Further, in many cases, the structural changes that can be detected are only rough approximations of brain injury as a whole. As noted previously, in many courtroom cases level of compensation rests mainly on functional changes. It is ironic that functional impairment is so important in so many courtroom cases, that neuropsychological assessment is often geared toward functional assessment and is a potential means for obtaining critical information, but that our measures tend to be modest, or even weak, predictors of everyday functioning (see Faust et al., 2011) and susceptible to manipulation. Important progress has been made in the assessment of function and considerable further gains are achievable, but the challenges will not be easy.

One way to view the appraisal of potential injury is as a task calling for a probability estimate, or as a type of base rate determination. In principle, the probability of injury ranges from 0% to 100%. In some cases, information is available that will all but rule out the occurrence of injury and help us to complete the task at hand.

Obviously, this will rarely be possible if the information we use to grade the likelihood of injury is not cumulatively valid and largely impervious to manipulation. Once the probabilities of injury exceed a certain level, however, we are back to a situation in which the second of the two basic determinations, in this case the occurrence of malingering, assumes critical relevance.

The effort to reach definitive or near-definitive judgments about injury and the resultant benefits that can accrue (e.g., no longer having to be particularly concerned about malingering when injury is absent) do not translate well to the appraisal of malingering. For example, even if we arguably could identify malingering with near certainty, it may help little (given current methods) in appraising the presence and severity of genuine injury. Furthermore, the cases in which we can rule out malingering with certainty or near certainty are likely to involve extreme presentations and occur infrequently. Thus, reaching a clear determination about malingering may not help much with the other side of the equation, which is appraising the presence and degree of genuine injury.

Research on the conjoint presentations of injury and malingering has certain elements in common with investigations of co-occurring conditions, but the parallels are incomplete and fortunately some of the worst methodological obstacles probably do not apply. Neuropsychological disorders or injuries and malingering probably have sufficient qualitative uniqueness that the problem of separating the two and measuring the relative presence of each is not intractable but at least partly solvable. Conceptually, it helps to distinguish the different ways variables may be related to a disorder and to malingering. Variables might: (a) not be valid or predictive in identifying either malingering or the injury in question; (b) show some degree of association with both dimensions; (c) show an association with one of the two but not the other; or (d) show a positive association with one and a negative association with the other. To illustrate these four classes of relationships: (a) certain demographic features might not relate to either malingering or the disorder in question; (b) decreased scores on measures of mental speed may show a similar strength of association with both; (c) anosmia may show a considerably stronger association with genuine disorder than it does with malingering; and (d) willingness to undergo painful medical treatments may show a positive association with injury and a negative association with malingering.

This list of potential relationships has a critical omission that is almost always highly relevant: variables that are also associated with other potential conditions or "rule outs." For example, suppose a variable shows a strong association with malingering, minimal association with head injury, but a strong association with, say, sleep disorder, and the latter is among the litigant's complaints or conditions and plausibly associated with the accident. As such, the variable will be of little or no use in separating out malingering and genuine disorder (in this case, sleep dysfunction). It is because litigants often present with a variety of complaints and possible conditions that promising results obtained in studies that exclude more complex presentations or alternative conditions may create a very misleading picture of success across applied settings. For the moment, however, we will focus on the first four classes of relationships and come back to this last concern later.

Given the problem under discussion—finding effective methods to evaluate the presence and degree of both malingering and injury—variables with no relation to either true injury or malingering are worthless, as are, at some level, variables that have about an equal association with each. (These latter variables can have value for other purposes, for example, if they help in separating one or both of these conditions from other alternatives.) If, in addition to all of the other things we are trying to accomplish through a forensic neuropsychological examination, we are attempting to determine the extent to which results are attributable to malingering and to true injury, a variable with a similar association to both does not move the inquiry forward. It is critically important to distinguish between variables that have a valid association with the conditions, as opposed to a subset of those variables, if present, that also help to differentiate the conditions or appraise their relative standing. No matter the degree of validity, if the variable changes to a similar extent when either malingering or injury is present, it will do us no good for these specific purposes. Thus, we seek variables that are both valid and *differentiating*.

Differentiating value is relative, not in the sense that evaluations of art may be relative to the perceiver or constructed, but relative to the task at hand. A variable that assists in distinguishing between, say, malingering versus head injury might not be at all effective in separating malingering from the effects of CO exposure at certain levels or duration. Therefore, the degree of differentiation possible is often specific to the particular conditions or tasks at hand. In many cases, it is a highly variable quality. The need for both validity and differentiating value, and the potential variations in differentiating value for different dimensions and situations make it all but a non sequitur to describe *the* validity of a malingering detection method, especially when phraseology is meant to convey accuracy. Obviously, accuracy is not a global quality and validity alone (e.g., association with malingering) is insufficient to make the needed determinations.

In contrast, if a variable has a greater degree of association with only malingering or with only the injury in question or, even better, if the variable is associated with both but the direction of association is reversed, it has differentiating value. We should look, first and foremost, for this latter or final class of variables but, to the extent we come up short, variables with different degrees of association with the two dimensions can certainly also have value. It should be apparent that studies failing to examine both validity and differentiating value will not suit our pragmatic needs. Furthermore, studies that merely establish an association between a variable and the presence or absence of one factor (either malingering or injury) will not help us here. Even if a variable shows a high association with malingering and consistently differentiates simulators from controls, it does us little or no good because we also need to know whether or how the variable is associated with true injury.

Most current test methods for appraising effort or malingering in the cognitive domain, to the extent they are effective, tend to work within an important but restricted domain. These methods usually examine for performance below expectation. Even when emphasis is placed on deviation from an expected pattern of results or on deficits in areas in which they are not expected, the final common path for detection of malingering is usually lowered performance. For example, if someone shows deficits (i.e., low scores) in areas in which one is not supposed to have deficits, this still comes down to a variation on the same theme—performing below expectation, whether this involves much poorer performances than are expected given the injury in question or the presence of deficits where there should not be deficits. There is nothing wrong in principle with this important detection strategy, but it is likely to be ineffectual in capturing other approaches malingerers might use to create misimpressions, such as false attribution or the provision of an exaggerated baseline. Although detection of underperformance may prove sufficient when a falsifier joins these or related strategies with diminished test effort, other fabricators may be sufficiently cagey to avoid gilding the lily and may limit themselves to misreporting. In such cases, most of our routine methods for assessing malingering, especially those restricted to cognitive measures, are likely to fail. For the moment, however, in order to approach the current topic systematically, we will focus on underperformance and methods designed to detect it.

The impact of malingering and true disorder on measures, such as test scores, can be additive, distinct, or interactive. To illustrate an *additive* relationship, assume someone's prior ability in an area of memory falls at a Wechsler-type scaled score equivalent of 100. If the individual is only injured (not malingering), the score might fall to 90; if only malingering (not injured), the resultant score might be 85; and if both injured and malingering, the score might fall to 80. To describe the relation as additive does not mean *strictly* additive, only that the combination produces a greater impact than either condition alone. Further, the proportionate contributions of one variable will not necessarily hold for another variable. Although malingering might account for, say, 80% of the change on one variable, it might account for a much smaller percentage on another variable.

Relationships for other variables might not be additive but *distinctive*. By distinctive, we mean that whatever the impact of either malingering or true injury on a variable, the other dimension will not exert an influence. For example, although malingering might reduce performance on a measure of overlearned material by a modest amount, true injury may have little or no impact on that variable. (In our initial description, we were presenting idealized types, but sometimes additive contributions will be so minor that for practical purposes the relation can usually be characterized as distinct without negative consequences.) Finally, *interactive* relationships obviously cannot occur without the presence of both malingering and true disorder.

For these three kinds of relationships, effects will not necessarily be limited to malingering and one particular condition, such as head injury. As follows, malingering may show additive, distinct, or interactive effects with other disorders or conditions that may also be present, some of which may be entirely independent of the event at issue; the same is true for injury or another condition under consideration. Given the range of potential influences on neuropsychological testing and the relative rarity with which these influences will be limited to malingering and a specific condition, beyond hypothetical cases or the unusually clean cases that might be selected for inclusion in research studies, one is usually dealing with a complex causal puzzle.

With these preliminaries in place, we can consider the manner in which detection strategies combine with various classes of relationship between malingering, genuine injury, and predictive variables. When the main detection strategy is directed at performance below expected levels, additive relationships between malingering and true injury increase the likelihood that the level of one or the other will be overidentified and may change these odds markedly. Furthermore, given the predisposition of some diagnosticians to view malingering and true injury as alternative possibilities as opposed to conjoint phenomena (they think too much "*or*" and too little "*and*"), the risk of false-negative errors in the identification of true injury or malingering (but not both simultaneously) may also increase. To the extent that true injury as opposed to malingering contributes to lower performance levels and moves one beyond cutting scores, overestimations of the role that malingering plays are likely to become more frequent, sizeable, and serious. Of particular concern, when injury alone is responsible for diminished capability, the least fortunate—those who fall at the negative end of the I+/M− continuum shown in Fig. 5—are most susceptible to false-positive errors in the identification of malingering and false-negative errors in the identification of injury. At the same time, these are the individuals who have the most to lose (i.e., they have already lost the most and may be most in need). Worries of this sort make the matter of combined presentations especially pressing, and ignoring the issue by concluding, for example, that one knows malingering is present and therefore cannot determine the extent to which true injury is present is not really a good default option. Rather, such a position is most likely to cause harm in cases in which there is an especially compelling moral obligation to avoid it.

When using performance below expectation as a detection strategy, one wants to separate the relative contributions (if any) of insufficient effort and true injury. A basic study design would compare the magnitude of impact on test performances for a group that is malingering but not injured, a group that is injured but not malingering, and a group that is both injured and malingering. A related design would start with an injured group and experimentally manipulate level of effort to examine the effects of such variation on results. One could also use designs that keep level of effort constant and use appropriate patient selection to vary level of injury.

Another approach, which might also start with a group that is malingering only and another that is injured only, would search for variables that achieve both validity and differentiating value. Such study designs have been used frequently with the aim of identifying variables that are likely to be altered by either true injury or malingering but not both. It is even better if one can find variables associated in opposite directions with injury and malingering. These study designs might be bolstered by also introducing groups in which malingering and injury are intermixed to varying degrees to examine the impact of conjoint presentations. For example, working with an injured group, one could experimentally manipulate level of effort. The goal is to determine if certain characteristics help separate the relative contributions of true injury and level of effort, with the long-term aim being the possible development of corrective methods or adjustments. Corrective methods or scales are commonly created for personality tests, and some of them, at least within certain ranges, demonstrate at least modest levels of efficacy. Little effort has been made to develop corrective methods for cognitive tests, perhaps because feigning is too often treated as a dichotomous variable or because measures are mainly designed to detect only grossly inadequate effort, both of which seem to have in common too much "or" versus "and" thinking.

Most alternative detection strategies depend on some sort of variation in expected performances (although some of these merge into methods aimed at underperformance). For example, one might look for deviation from expected course over time, atypical symptoms such as the co-presentation of complaints that usually do not co-occur (e.g., a report of anosmia but heightened smell sensation at other times), or deviation from expected highs and lows in test scores. Most such strategies depend on identifying outcome variables that are distinctive (minimally overlap across the injured and those who are malingering) and which thereby may provide both validity and differentiating value. Here again, one can compare individuals who are malingering and not injured to a group that is injured and not malingering, and also implement designs in which level of injury varies and level of effort is experimentally manipulated.

The situation is much more complicated when the impact of injury and malingering interact, and the end result may not be lower performance relative to common levels when individuals are malingering but not injured. For example, someone with true injury may not feel the need to alter performance more than a little to achieve adequate recognition of impairment and may be conservative in these efforts rather than risk being viewed as entirely fraudulent. In other situations, interactions lead to performance below expected levels for either condition alone. We do not mean to play armchair philosopher and only wish to make two points. First, anticipating interactive effects is often very difficult and best determined through formal study. Second, one thing that is fairly certain is that the majority of interactive effects will alter test patterns.

We mention this matter of pattern alteration with trepidation because we fear it could be mistaken for the argument that such determinations should rest primarily on clinical judgment and that the analysis should involve the integration of many variables and the attempt to discern complex interrelationships. We are not arguing for either of these positions and believe they are more counterproductive than constructive (see the prior discussion of interpretive strategies). Rather, fairly simple and much more psychometrically sound methods can be used to appraise deviation from expectation. Suppose one identified a composite of variables that were more likely to be impacted by head injury than by malingering and another composite that were more likely to be impacted by malingering. Within each composite, the results might be calculated for each component variable by measuring distance from expectation (for that variable) and then summing across the variables. The first cumulative index might assist in judging the likelihood that test scores were impacted by head injury and the second the likelihood that scores were impacted by malingering, with a possible supplemental procedure used to estimate the relative contributions of the two indexes. Variation from expectation does not require complex pattern analysis, and simple linear composites of deviation measurements might be quite effective and easily quantifiable, thereby reducing dependence on subjective judgment.

Obstacles Created by *Inter-* and *Intra-*Individual Variation and the Need for Baseline Measurement

Even if methods are used that enhance psychometric quality (such as linear composites to increase reliability), approaches emphasizing performance below expected level or deviation from expected performance patterns will almost surely fall far short of their true promise if limited to contemporaneous measurement. Absent sufficient information about baseline functioning, *inter-* and *intra-*individual variation will often overwhelm disorder-specific effects, which is a major problem not only in malingering detection but for almost any form of pattern analysis in neuropsychology, especially approaches emphasizing more than rudimentary configurations.

As is well known, *inter-*individual variation refers to the distribution in performance across individuals. Even within normal samples or those with no known pathology, performance ranges in many areas are extreme. For example, the difference between, say, a 40-year-old who obtains a borderline versus a very superior score on the WAIS-IV Information subtest is 3–4 correct answers versus 23 correct answers (Wechsler, 2008). *Intra-*individual variation refers to an individual's range or "scatter" in scores across areas and is frequently much greater than is commonly assumed. As has been known for decades, normal individuals will often show large differences in performance across areas, especially as the number of administered tests expands (e.g., Binder, Iverson, & Brooks, 2009; Brooks, Iverson, Sherman, & Holdnack, 2009; Brooks, Strauss, Sherman, Iverson, & Slick, 2009; Cook et al., 2019; Dumont & Willis, 1995; Schretlen, Munro, Anthony, & Pearlson, 2003; Schretlen & Sullivan, 2013). For example, even in circumstances that, if anything, tended to reduce intra-individual variation (e.g., co-norming and a modest versus high number of tests), Schretlen et al. (2003) obtained a mean difference between normal individuals' highest and lowest scores of 3.4 standard deviations (SD), with 20% of the sample obtaining differences of 4 SD or more.

By *disorder-specific effects,* we mean true differential impact of diseases or conditions on functions. Suppose, for example, that moderate head injury causes a mean decline of 1.0 SD in new visual memory, .5 SD in delayed verbal recall, and .1 SD or less in some area of overlearned factual knowledge. Disorder-specific effects have a true magnitude, but measurements of these effects are approximations with varying error terms that, unfortunately, are often disturbingly large for reasons we will touch on momentarily. Different conditions or disorders are likely to have partly or largely overlapping disorder-specific effects, making the term somewhat of an oxymoron. However, what we are referring to is the adverse impact of the condition or event in question and not unique effects in relation to all other conditions and disorders that can alter neuropsychological functioning.

When attempting to differentiate a normal individual from one afflicted with a specific disorder, one does not worry about overlap with other disorders; but when one must distinguish among possible disorders or combinations of disorders—probably the more usual situation in neuropsychology—overlap in the effects produced by disorders can become a major concern. As the number of possible conditions or disorders that must be considered expands (e.g., are viable possibilities) and as the degree of overlap increases, distinctions become more difficult. This is one reason it may be considerably more difficult to sort out malingering and injury than malingering versus normality, especially when litigants may also be impacted by multiple other conditions or factors. The difference between a disorder-specific effect and normality, on average, is greater or far greater than the difference between two disorders and conditions that can both impact neuropsychological functioning. For example, although a moderate-to-severe head injury may cause an average difference of 1.5 SD between those with and without such injury in a certain area of functioning, the contrast may be much smaller between those so injured and those feigning deficit and may run in the reverse direction (e.g., performance averaging .5 SD lower for the malingering group).

Given their relative magnitudes, the impact of intra- and inter-individual variation on test performance often overwhelms the influence of disorder-specific factors, especially when one is not so concerned with separating normal individuals from others but rather must undertake more complex differentials. For example, if testing is normal, there is often little left to do. However, when testing is abnormal, one will commonly be faced with a differential involving both malingering and injury, and often will also need to evaluate the potential impact of additional possibilities (e.g., mood disorder, a history of prior head injury, substance use/abuse). The more subtle or less robust distinguishing features are, then to the extent error enters into the analysis due to inter- and intra-individual variation, the greater the diagnostic problem and likelihood of getting it wrong. Inter- and intra-individual variation can be viewed almost as error components (like variation within groups when one is comparing across groups in studies) and may exert much greater effects than disorder-specific effects given the methods of analysis that are routine in clinical and forensic practice.

These abstractions can be concretized through graphic representation, starting with somewhat extreme exemplars for the sake of clarity. Figure 6 depicts inter-individual variation for a specific function, say, mental speed. Presume a test used to measure this function has a mean of 100 and a standard deviation of 15. The pre-event standing of two hypothetical individuals, Smith and Jones, fall toward opposite ends of the performance continuum, but not at pre-injury levels that extend more than 2 standard deviations beyond the mean. Assume that Smith and Jones both experience mild head injuries and are later tested with a battery that includes this measure of mental speed. Assume the respective neuropsychologists who examine either Smith or Jones do not have knowledge of prior abilities in this area, or that Smith and Jones had never been tested before the accident. Thus, their baselines in Fig. 6 represent their true prior capacities, but these are unknown quantities. (We recognize that relative extremes in prior abilities should not be missed.)

Suppose an investigator has studied the effect of comparable head injuries on this measure. When compared to matched controls, the injured group demonstrates a mean decline of .70 standard deviations, or about 10 points, and few injured individuals exhibit a decline of more than 20 points. Thus, a score below 80 is sufficiently unusual among the study sample that it is suggested for use as a cutoff for identifying insufficient effort. The exact figures we set forth in this hypothetical are

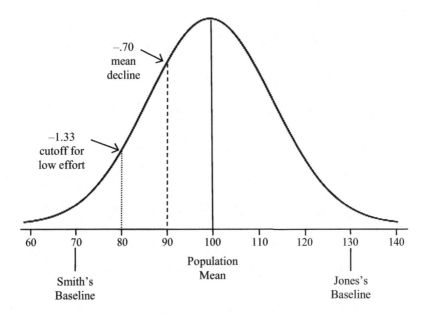

Fig. 6 *Inter*-individual variation vs. disorder-specific decrements, using mental speed as an example

not important as our main intent is illustrative, but they are not unrealistic. In studies of standard neuropsychological tests, such results would not be outlandish, nor the suggestion that performances this far below expectation could be considered a possible indicator of falsification. Even should one set the cutoff at a different level, the relative impact on overall error will be similar and will merely change the relative frequencies of false-positive and false-negative error; for example, if one sets a more stringent cutting point to reduce the risk of false-positive error, the rate of false-negative error will increase.

Figure 7 demonstrates the detrimental effects of inter-individual variation on classification accuracy when the obtained cutting score is applied. Smith's injury has produced a drop in his mental speed that translates into a 10 point loss on the measure. He is also making his best effort on testing. Thus, he is injured and not malingering. Nevertheless, he will be identified as putting forth insufficient effort on the measure. He becomes saddled with a false-positive identification of malingering, and his injury might also be missed, an unfortunate false-negative error. We have plotted two possible results for Jones. If Jones is injured and malingering, both are likely to be missed. If Jones is injured and not malingering, then although he at least will probably not be misidentified as a fabricator, his true injury is likely to be missed.

Although Smith and Jones fall at far ends of the continuum, there is a large range of above average (pre-event) ability levels that creates a considerable risk of false-negative error for injury and a large range of below average (pre-event) ability levels that creates a considerable risk of false-positive error for malingering. Furthermore,

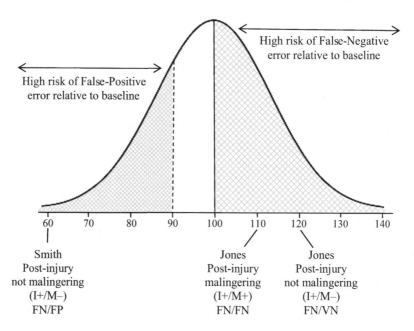

Fig. 7 Impact of *inter*-individual variability on false-positive (FP) and false-negative (FN) error rates

for those with above average abilities, there is considerable risk that true injury will be missed (with a corresponding increase in the false-positive error rate for those with below average abilities). Therefore, it is not only at the extremes of the continuum for which the risk of error is great when evaluating both malingering and injury status but also for large proportions of the distribution, all due to inter-individual variation.

Sociodemographically adjusted norms may help somewhat in reducing the impact of inter-individual variation, but often less than is commonly assumed. First, methods that emphasize performance below expected levels on standard tests may not use demographically adjusted scores, hence leading to exactly the sort of problem illustrated in Fig. 7. An equal or greater problem starts with both formal and informal methods for estimating prior functioning, but it is too involved to describe comprehensively in the present work. The notion is to adjust expectation for performance based on knowledge of baseline functioning. Thus, if one knows a person was very capable prior to the accident, expectations for performance (and for identifying performance that raises concerns about cooperation) are modified, as would be the case with someone with low prior capabilities, although in the first case expectations are raised and in the latter case lowered. The limits of using impressionistic methods to estimate prior functioning have been pointed out in the literature, in particular their susceptibility to substantial error (e.g., Faust & Ahern, 2011; Kareken & Williams, 1994; Williams, 1998). With formal methods, whether explicitly stated or not, the main thrust is often the prediction of overall intellectual ability.

The problem this creates is that overall ability may not be a strong predictor of other variables assessed during neuropsychological evaluation.

The extent to which neuropsychological assessment enhances or improves upon intellectual assessment alone depends on the independence or nonredundancy of the two methods. If neuropsychological measures correlated too highly with intellectual testing, they would not provide unique or nonredundant information. Hence, the extent to which neuropsychological tests contribute above and beyond intellectual testing rests not only on their validity but also on their degree of independence from intellectual measures and is one of the most basic rationales for the entire enterprise. All else being equal, the greater the independence the greater the extent to which accuracy is increased; that is, the greater the contribution of neuropsychological evaluation to incremental validity. The obverse side of this psychometric fundamental is that attributes that make neuropsychological measures most effective (by maximizing their independence from intellectual testing and hence their contribution to incremental validity) all but ensure that whatever best predicts intellectual testing results will not best predict results on these same neuropsychological measures. If A (a Full Scale IQ score) is minimally related to B (a specific neuropsychological test result), and if C is a strong (or maximal) predictor of A, then C cannot be a strong predictor of B as well. Measures that best predict prior intelligence will often be weak or poor predictors of the neuropsychological tests that are most sensitive to brain injuries or contribute the most to incremental validity, and thus if methods for determining prior functioning mainly address intelligence, they are likely to be unsatisfactory predictors of these neuropsychological measures.

Adjustments for sociodemographic factors (in effect, a way of narrowing the comparison group and thereby attempting to better approximate prior functioning) are generally geared toward overall intellectual functioning and thus are much more effective predictors of that quality than of specific areas of neuropsychological functioning. The end result is that sociodemographic adjustment or other methods that directly or indirectly estimate prior functioning often do not do much to adjust for inter-individual (or intra-individual) variation in specific areas of neuropsychological functioning. For example, even if an individual is compared to other individuals with fairly similar levels of intellectual ability, this often does not go that far in assuring similarity in other areas of neuropsychological functioning, especially those areas that are least redundant with intelligence and most sensitive to brain damage or yield the highest levels of incremental validity.

Additionally, knowing an individual's general level of intellectual ability does not help much with the problems created by intra-individual variability. Figure 8 shows Smith having a true pre-event mental speed score of 70 and a true new learning capacity score of 130. Such variation is not rare (see Schretlen et al., 2003), although in one way we have represented a worst-case scenario because this large intra-individual contrast happens to occur across two areas that are often both affected by head injuries. Suppose again that the cutoff score for poor effort is 80, that the injury has adversely affected Smith's mental speed but not his new learning, and that in the latter area Smith is feigning deficit. Due to the combination of baseline functioning and true loss, Smith's mental speed score falls far below the cutoff

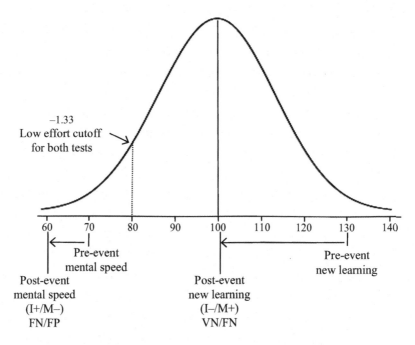

Fig. 8 Illustration of impact of *intra*-individual vs. disorder-specific decrements

for malingering. Consequently, the true injury is missed (a false-negative error) and malingering is falsely identified (a false-positive error). Ironically, in the area of new learning, where he has grossly underperformed due to malingering alone, the absence of any effect from injury is identified correctly (a valid-negative judgment) but malingering is missed (a false-negative error). In fact, Smith would have had to score at least 10 points *above* his pre-injury baseline in mental speed not to be falsely identified as a malingerer, and more than 50 points *below* his true new learning baseline to be detected as malingering in that area. Consequently, although the scenario presented here represents one of the worst problems that can result from intra-individual variation, less extreme occurrences, which are common, can easily lead to errors. More generally, whether using general population norms, impressionistic methods, or formal techniques that are currently available to try to account for baseline functioning, inter- and intra-individual variation will often overpower or overwhelm disorder-specific effects and lead to frequent errors.

We would go a long way toward eliminating the error component caused by inter- and intra-individual variability with even brief and routine population baseline assessments of neuropsychological functioning. Such information would be invaluable beyond malingering assessment. The tremendous advantages of systematically implemented pre-injury testing are being demonstrated in such areas as sports-related injury (although sometimes not as well as might be given the psychometric limits of some approaches), and we hope that a broader lesson can be drawn from such examples. If neuropsychologists can get on board with reducing the length of neuropsychological testing—at least for baseline screening—through such methods as adaptive testing, and continue increasing the use of computer technology, it may be possible in coming years to implement broad-based population screening. For example, a 30-min screen administered every decade in widely used healthcare settings could be of great personal and social benefit and advance the field remarkably.

Neuropsychologists are leery about recommendations to shorten their test batteries, and there are certainly times when truncating assessment due to external pressure rather than best practices is damaging. Even when prioritizing incremental validity, if multiple decision points need to be addressed and cumulative indices are among the most effective predictors but require fairly lengthy testing, relatively long batteries may be needed to approach a ceiling in effectiveness. However, when the purpose is population-based screening, such lengthy procedures are often impractical, inefficient, and excessive, and if we continue to insist on them there is little chance of accomplishing this worthy aim. A method solely aimed at a single determination, which is whether there is an unacceptably high probability that an anomalous decline in overall functioning or on a cumulative index has occurred, could serve an essential decision-making purpose, which is to differentiate those who do and do not need more comprehensive evaluation. (A main challenge here is overcoming limits in successive hurdles approaches or in developing the psychometric refinements needed to make screening truly effective, as discussed earlier in the volume.) It may also be shortsighted to assume that reducing length will have a negative long-term economic impact, because almost surely the opposite outcome would result. Imagine if years ago individuals meeting in an IBM conference room agreed that cutting the cost of computers would be bad financial policy. Even if such a policy was financially neutral or negative, which it probably is not, improvement in patient care should be the determining factor.

A higher aspiration is to address questions through baseline assessment that go beyond "stop-go" decisions about those who do and do not need further evaluation. By following psychometric principles carefully, a surprising amount might be accomplished in a relatively short period of time. The availability of an earlier or pre-event baseline could make major contributions to clinical and legal assessments. For example, in legal cases, it could greatly facilitate attempts to determine whether adverse change has occurred following a mild head injury, especially if evaluation of effort improves in tandem. Our techniques for estimating pre-injury functioning are so limited at present that even modest success in baseline assessment would improve our situation considerably.

In designing screens with future comparisons in mind, targets might include more frequently occurring conditions that are generally more difficult to identify without a pre-post comparison and for which early identification can reap maximum benefit. For example, the early identification of dementia or its functional consequences, given anticipated improvements in our capacity for helpful intervention, might well be one such target condition. One would likely focus on relatively non-redundant areas in which the greatest changes occur on average, adding items one at a time that make a unique and maximal contribution to incremental validity.

When distinguishing between one and another condition is critical, one would focus on variables that have the joint qualities of validity and differentiating value. By measuring and updating appraisal of baseline or pre-event functioning, one can reduce or nearly eliminate two of the biggest sources of error for many forms of neuropsychological evaluation, inter- and intra-individual variation. (We understand, of course, that evaluation of intra-individual variation can serve other critical purposes in neuropsychological evaluation.)

In the meantime, while waiting for these hoped for advances, those wishing to evaluate deviation from expected performance levels must do their best with what is available. It would seem evident that current approaches for postdicting pre-event functioning using contemporaneous measures and perhaps sociodemographic variables that are aimed at intellectual functioning have limited utility. Studies on these approaches tend to be restricted to examining the accuracy with which overall intellectual indices can be determined, and we have noted the limited relation that often holds between general intellectual functioning and the more specific measures that add the most to the diagnostic power of neuropsychological assessment. If one wants a sobering look at how poorly such methods seem to work for predicting functioning in specific areas, Schretlen, Buffington, Meyer, and Pearlson's study (2005) provides an instructive example. In essence, one is using a variable (A) to predict intellectual functioning (B) in order to predict functioning in specific areas (C), despite knowing that B often shows limited association with C. The result is to multiply error: predictive power is lost by introducing an additional inferential link (using A to predict B to predict C), and one is using B to predict C despite knowing that they often do not show a strong association.

If one is going to attempt these approaches, it is much more advantageous to predict C directly from A, by identifying variables that predict functioning in specific areas. For example, with the typical approach, one identifies a combination of variables that correlate with a prior Full Scale IQ score (FSIQ). These composite variables might achieve a correlation in the .50s. One then uses the estimated FSIQ score to predict, say, the capacity for new visual learning, which may show a correlation of .40 with FSIQ. This obviously degrades predictive capacity severely; if A correlates with B at .50, but B correlates with C at .40, then the ultimate power to predict C is poor. In contrast, if some combination of variables shows a correlation of, say .30 with C, then by avoiding the extra inferential link this obtained level, although considerably weaker than the original association between the other predictive variables and FSIQ (i.e., between A and B), is still likely to be a stronger predictor.

In principle, so long as neuropsychological measures are assessing functions with reasonable degrees of reliability, prior standing in those areas should be as predictable as, say, overall intelligence. For example, if we have a measure of visual memory with a .85 reliability, that level might not be quite as good as it is for FSIQ, but it still gives us a decent chance to identify predictors with at least a modest level of accuracy. In contrast, if measures of specific functions have relatively weak or poor reliability, as is sometimes the case with neuropsychological tests and especially subcomponent scores (e.g., some of the variables that might be examined on a word list learning test), then the prospects for even modestly effective postdiction is poor. It is almost a given, considering the relatively low correlations between FSIQ and various neuropsychological tests, as well as the modest to low correlations often obtained among neuropsychological tests themselves, that the best postdictors will often vary from test to test, and sometimes considerably. For example, if new visual learning correlates minimally with finger tapping speed, there is almost no chance that the same set of predictors will optimize postdiction of both functions. This is why normative systems that adjust along the same set of sociodemographic variables for all tests, although an important start, have very different degrees of success across measures and will not come close to optimizing postdiction or optimal comparison on a test-by-test basis. Rather, the daunting task, if one were to fully pursue this approach, is to identify the most effective predictors idiosyncratically, or separately for each measure. The consequences of uneven success rates produced by sociodemographic adjustment wreaks havoc with pattern analysis yet is rarely mentioned, operating below the surface or perhaps without full recognition of what is occurring.

Given all of the limits and complexities involved in using contemporaneous tests to determine prior functioning, one is often better off accessing previously obtained measures. Even here, there is a very limited data base on the relation between measures that are commonly used in schools or other settings (e.g., the workplace, the military) and performance on specific neuropsychological measures as opposed to more general measures of intellectual aptitude or academic achievement, and a number of cautions need to be implemented (see Baade & Schoenberg, 2004; Orme, Ree, & Rioux, 2001; Reynolds, 1997; Williams, 1997).

Finally, and perhaps an unsettling thought, the co-occurrence of malingering and injury, which adds considerable complexities to forensic neuropsychological evaluation and research challenges, is only a component of many presentations. Additional factors—some causally related to the event in question and some that are not, and some that occupy critical links in the causal chain but that may be subtle, indirect, or multiple steps removed from the original event—all may impede effort or diminish test performance. Consequently, all might impact on predominant methods for assessing malingering, which rest on performance below expected levels or deviation from expected patterns (e.g., atypical symptoms, atypical course). For example, a car accident may cause orthopedic injuries that cause pain and reduced ability to bear weight. These problems may in turn diminish activity and, when combined with medication side effects, lead to weight gain over the course of months, which produces sleep apnea, which diminishes cognitive functioning and motivation. Many research studies are exercises in oversimplification, which can be necessary or helpful for certain purposes, but which may fail to capture the clinician's real world to such an extent that the findings are misleading and result in frequent error when applied directly. In many forensic cases, there may be at least a half dozen causal factors to consider when appraising neuropsychological status and effort, and this is why it is often only the extreme cases (e.g., definitely not injured, or having overwhelming injury) that are clear-cut but for which the neuropsychologist's expertise may be least needed.

Mixed Presentations: Some Additional Thoughts

As a starting point, it can be very helpful to sort injury and effort into dichotomous categories. Unless dichotomous classification is performed properly, attempts at greater refinement are doomed from the start. When either or both are present, a next step can be to determine degree. If both are present and degree can be measured, it may be possible, at least under some circumstances, to adjust measurement of injury in relation to level of effort. For example, it might be possible to develop methods to regress test scores in relation to level of effort. Such corrective methods are likely to be feasible only within a certain range of effort. For example, effort might be so poor that true level of capacity cannot be determined, much as would be the case if an individual responded to every item on a personality questionnaire by providing the deviant answer. It is unrealistic to believe that these difficult determinations can be made routinely and with a high degree of accuracy without formal scientific help and properly validated decision rules, and thus the burden falls on researchers to continue the impressive track record of success and to push the boundaries of knowledge a good deal further. It is as much mistaken to undervalue what has been accomplished as it is to believe that we are all that close to a perfect solution.

When examining for performance below expectation, measures specifically designed to assess malingering often produce much greater differences between those who are injured and those who are malingering than do standard neuropsychological tests. The degree of separation these specialized methods create may foster much greater accuracy in dichotomous classification than standard measures achieve. For one, additional factors that diminish effort, such as marked anxiety, may not impact results on the specialized tests very much. Many of the specialized measures are deceptively easy and thus are often insensitive to true injury or conditions that alter results on standard neuropsychological measures. In contrast, many neuropsychological tests are designed to be sensitive to cognitive dysfunction (of numerous potential kinds or causes) and, therefore, scores on them will often be diminished not only by malingering but also by dozens of other factors related to true organic or functional malady. Additionally, because specialized tests may create large differences in the first place, even if modest alterations do occur secondary to other variables, overall classifications will frequently remain unaltered. For example, in studies at least, the difference between the injured and the malingerers might be about three standard deviations for a specialized test and one standard deviation for a traditional neuropsychological test. Thus, for example, if a moderate-to-severe mood disorder lowers performance on both the malingering measure and a standard neuropsychological measure by about three-fourths of a standard deviation, it will minimally impact the malingering test yet all but obliterate accuracy for the standard test.

It is this positive quality of specialized malingering tests, however, that has yielded a consequence that is likely to greatly compromise their potential for appraising the degree of malingering, especially when it is not extreme, and thereby their potential for assisting in the design and calculation of corrective indices. The separations may be so good that distributions are highly skewed and relatively few errors are required to place an examinee into an extreme class. One result is that once one exceeds thresholds for poor effort, there may be very little room for variation in test scores. For example, on one popular malingering test, anything below 90% accurate responses can be highly suggestive of poor effort. However, this measure and most others like it are designed to detect extreme departures from good cooperation, and passing them does not mean an individual has necessarily exerted even a modest level of effort, much less a high or optimum level. As a result, scores below cutoff points can be very helpful in identifying poor effort, but scores above them may leave only a few items and a very small range of differing results. Given such truncated ranges for "passing" scores, there is little chance that relative level of effort, or varying degrees of suboptimal effort, can be distinguished or that results could serve a corrective function. Such a limitation, which in no way is intended as a criticism of specialized malingering tests that were designed for other purposes, could be addressed in various ways. For example, one could add branching procedures that increase the item pool and produce a wider range of possible scores, or simply add other measures that may be more effective in assessing relative levels of effort.

5.2 The Extreme Group Problem

A central theme of this volume is the importance of focusing research efforts on ambiguous cases. The cases with which practitioners need help are not the definitive or near-definitive (D/ND) presentations but cases involving closer calls, in which it appears as if someone might be malingering but the matter is not that clear-cut. This is the group suspected of malingering, some of whom are indeed malingering and some of whom are not.

It is to the credit of researchers that the percentage of ambiguous cases has steadily declined, although the proportion that remains may be a good deal larger than is sometimes thought due to the more complex determinations that are commonly necessary, such as joint consideration of injury status and malingering. An important additional factor in underestimations of ambiguous cases is what we have labeled the *extreme group problem* (EGP). Stated succinctly, participants in studies often overrepresent more clear-cut cases (D/ND malingerers and D/ND nonmalingerers) in comparison to the more subtle or ambiguous presentations that create greater clinical challenges. Inclusion of these more extreme cases in turn creates a host of problems, including qualitative and quantitative distortions in research outcomes that frequently undermine generalization and clinical applicability.

Cohen (1988, 1992) subdivided effect sizes into small (0.2), medium (0.5), and large (0.8), not as hard and fast demarcation points but as an interpretive aid. Keeping these proposed classifications in mind, one can ask what is wrong with effect sizes like the following:

4.20	4.57	5.30	8.14
4.23	4.65	5.47	10.24
4.42	4.76	5.74	10.38
4.49	4.90	6.53	13.66

The first and obvious answer is that they are highly implausible and that true differences of this magnitude are almost never obtained in applied psychology. The second and disturbing answer, however, is that they are among the effect sizes reported for scales F and Fb in a meta-analysis of malingering detection with the MMPI-2 (Rogers, Sewell, Martin, & Vitacco, 2003). We are not faulting the authors in any way because they are merely reporting the outcomes of studies, but the fact that effect sizes in this range were obtained in over 10% of results reported across studies in this meta-analysis is concerning. In another meta-analysis of malingering detection (Vickery, Berry, Inman, Harris, & Orey, 2001), effect sizes for two commonly used measures exceeded 4.00 for 15% of the outcomes. A naïve reader of the literature might take such figures literally and form a grossly overblown impression about diagnostic accuracy in real-life application. Obviously, something is seriously amiss, and what is amiss is the EGP. What these highly implausible effect sizes do not reveal is how much more pervasive the EGP is in areas of psychology and especially in research on malingering detection.

The Rogers et al. (2003) MMPI-2 meta-analysis lists 78 study outcomes or effect sizes for the F scale and 51 effect sizes for the Fb scale. Figure 9 tallies the number and percentage of effect sizes for these two scales that exceeded 1.00. If we take effect sizes of 1.00–1.99 as pushing the boundaries of plausibility, 2.00–2.99 as highly questionable, and 3.00 or greater as very likely implausible, one finds that for the F scale nearly 7 out of 10 effects sizes (69%) push or exceed the boundaries of plausibility, and more than half (54%) are highly questionable or implausible. For the 51 effect sizes for Fb, 65% push the bounds of plausibility and nearly half are highly questionable or implausible (i.e., ES = 2.00 or greater). The situation is even more extreme for some of the measures included in the Vickery et al. (2001) meta-analysis. Figure 9 also provides the combined results (designated as *Vickery*) for the Digit Memory Test and the Portland Digit Recognition Test. For these two tests together, *100% of the outcomes* push or exceed the boundaries of plausibility, and 65% (i.e., those exceeding 2.00) are highly questionable or implausible.

Our interpretations are not intended to criticize the authors of the meta-analyses or to imply that the measures do not have value. For example, an effect size of, say. 1.0 can reflect a truly robust measure with strong psychometric or predictive properties. Furthermore, even if an effect size is implausibly high, it does not mean that the true or intrinsic validity of the measure is not a contributor to the result. For example, the inflated outcome may be an effect size of 3.75, but the "true" effect size may still be a robust .80. (The word *true* is used in quotes because, of course, effect sizes vary with application, and the term is intended to reference the true value for the intended application.) What we do think is abundantly clear is that many of these

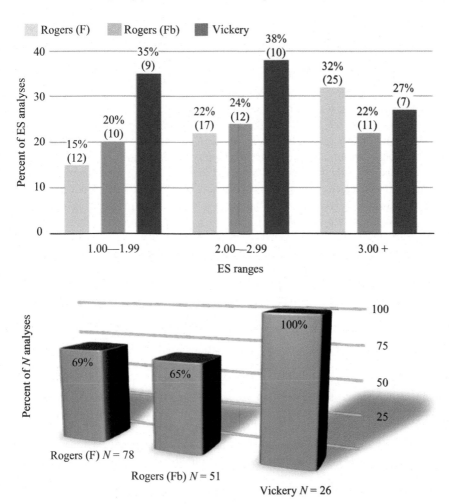

Fig. 9 Effect sizes exceeding 1.00 found in meta-analyses by Rogers et al. (2003; MMPI-2 scales F and Fb) and by Vickery et al. (2001) by size category (top) and for all ES analyses. (Percentages at top do not total to 100% for the Rogers et al. analyses because ES's below 1.00 are not included here; all of Vickery et al.'s ES's were 1.00 or greater.)

effect sizes are inflated, often by a sizeable amount, and that the problem is pervasive. This is, we believe, the EGP rearing its ugly head.

Explanation of the EGP

The EGP is a subtle and often underappreciated, but potent, methodological flaw that distorts the outcomes of studies and leads to inflated effect sizes. The degree of inflation can be extreme and lead to gross overestimation of effectiveness in the settings of intended application, such as forensic neuropsychological assessment in civil litigation. The EGP is by no means limited to research on malingering and occurs in numerous other assessment domains (see Bridges, Faust, & Ahern, 2009; Faust, Bridges, & Ahern, 2009a, 2009b), but its impact seems to be especially pernicious in malingering assessment.

For the moment, we can designate those suspected of malingering as MS, and further subdivide this group into those who are and are not malingering, respectively represented as MS+ (suspected and malingering) and MS− (suspected but not malingering). Presumably, malingering is suspected because of some departure from regularity, such as lower than expected scores on one or more standard neuropsychological measures. In research studies, the EGP is usually produced by the methods used to select both the malingering and the nonmalingering groups. In many cases, selection procedures for both groups result in overly extreme cases. The malingering group is more extreme than the typical MS+ case, with the difference representing more extreme cases of malingering. The control group's deviation is usually in the other direction, that is, they are more normal or unremarkable than the MS− group. Thus, both research groups are more extreme than typical cases but in opposing directions: the malingering group is more deviant than the MS+ group and the control or comparison group is less deviant (or more normal) than the MS− group.

One might ask why group selection procedures would permit this type of nonrepresentativeness to occur. Understandably, when selecting members for the malingering group, the researcher wants to be fairly certain that group members are malingering. Hence it is common to use fairly stringent inclusionary criteria that require markedly deviant results, such as clearly elevated scores on multiple malingering tests. Conversely, the researcher also seeks reassurance that those in the control group are not malingering, in which case fairly stringent inclusionary criteria might be set in the other direction. Here, one might require clean results on malingering tests and perhaps certain minimal scores on standard tests, or even status in a group (e.g., nonlitigants) in which incentives to malinger are limited or negligible. Ironically, one is therefore selecting individuals for whom there is little reason to suspect they are *not* malingering (the experimental group) and others for whom there is little reason to suspect they *are* malingering (the control group) to learn how to identify those whom we suspect are malingering and are malingering (the MS+ group) and those we suspect are malingering and are not malingering (the MS− group). If simulation designs are used, similar problems may occur, if for no other reason than a group of normal individuals who perform their best will often be markedly more normal or intact or neuropsychologically superior in comparison to the MS− group.

Evidence suggests that the EGP, or the magnitude of this methodological flaw, frequently accounts for far more variance in the outcomes of studies than the intrinsic or true quality of tests or assessment methods. If the numerous exceedingly high effect sizes in various meta-analyses are accounted for primarily by the EGP and these effects sizes may be inflated by a factor of two or three (or more), then clearly the EGP is the most influential determinant of outcome. We are obviously in a very bad methodological situation if the worse the design flaw, the better a method performs in studies, especially if the presence or magnitude of the EGP is underappreciated or not recognized. When there is a *positive* association between the degree of methodological flaw and the level of accuracy studies yield, we can be driven further and further from verisimilitude or the correct appraisal of methods.

In addition, if we are comparing different tests or assessment methods and the background studies do not overlap sufficiently, as is very commonly the case in malingering detection research, relative merits can be skewed or grossly distorted. Suppose test A is truly much better than test B. However, suppose further that the studies on test A are minimally saddled with the EGP, but that a separate set of studies on test B show this problem to a marked degree. As a consequence, accuracy rates or effect sizes generated for test B may seem much more favorable than those generated for test A. As we will later show through example, this sort of situation is not an abstraction because non-overlapping studies are common, even in meta-analyses, and have the potential to alter or even reverse rank ordering of efficacy. Consequently, even highly conscientious neuropsychologists who carefully incorporate scientific literature into their practices may be inadvertently led into making mistaken choices.

To illustrate the potential for distorted ranking due to non-overlapping studies, we can momentarily turn back to the Rogers et al. (2003) meta-analysis of MMPI-2 malingering scales or indices. As we noted, 78 effect sizes were reported for the F scale and 51 for the Fb scale. For almost every study involving Fb, results were also reported for F (50 of 51 analyses), something explained by the predominance of the F scale as an MMPI-2 malingering indicator. Thus, in 50 cases, the study groups were the same for F and Fb, thereby holding the EGP constant. For example, if a study examined effect sizes for Fb for two groups of subjects, the same two groups were used to calculate effect sizes for F as well. Whatever the magnitude of the EGP in those analyses, it was the same for both groups. There are different ways to summarize the results of the meta-analyses for these same-groups comparisons, and we will focus on a simple indicator for illustrative purposes.

For the same-groups analyses, 78% of the effect sizes exceeded 1.00 for F and 74% for Fb, suggesting that when the EGP is held constant the F scale might be a slightly stronger malingering indicator than Fb. This is not to say that the obtained effect sizes reflect applied performance, but if the EGP is held constant, then the relative efficacy of indicators or tests should not be altered or distorted (although other complications can arise that blur comparisons, such as differences in performance characteristic in relation to the standing of cases on the variables under study). Of interest, in the 28 non-overlapping studies—those that examined only F—54% of the effect sizes exceed 1.00, a considerably lower figure than the 78% obtained in the same-groups analyses. It is likely this lower rate was obtained because on average the non-overlapping studies have less extreme groups in comparison to the same-groups analyses. In the Rogers et al. meta-analysis, summary figures are provided for F and Fb, the former of which is a composite of the 50 same-group analyses and the 28 non-overlapping studies. Given the lower effect sizes for the F scale found in the non-overlapping analyses, the composite figure derived by combining the non-overlapping analyses and the same-groups analyses is 69%. Thus, in the same-groups studies in which the EGP is held constant, F slightly outperforms Fb (78–74%), but if one only reports the composite of the non-overlapping studies and same-group analyses it now appears as if Fb outperforms F (74–69%). This meta-analysis and these scales are used for illustrative purposes, and sometimes the contrasts between same-groups analyses and non-overlapping studies are far larger than the results obtained here.

It may be surprising how often meta-analyses do not show complete overlap across studies on tests or indicators, and in many cases the overlap may be limited or minimal. For example, in the Vickery et al. (2001) meta-analysis, which rank orders methods, there is minimal overlap in studies across a number of the indicators. Thus, it is difficult to discern the extent to which differences are a product of true contrasts in efficacy versus inconsistencies in the magnitude of the EGP (or across other variables). If, as we think is the case, the EGP frequently accounts for more variance than any other factor, and if the magnitude of the EGP may differ markedly across studies of various indicators or tests, then *rank orders may be far off and even negatively correlated with true values*.

The inflated accuracy rates the EGP produces are likely to lead in turn to over-confidence in malingering assessment methods. In earlier materials (see the section on "Overconfidence"), we detailed the multiple adverse consequences that can result from inflated confidence, such as reduced accuracy and an increased tendency to make overly risky and harmful decisions. Furthermore, to the extent the EGP distorts the relative ranking of tests or procedures, it can easily lead to nonoptimal or poor selection of methods. For example, a test with a true error rate of 40% might be selected over one with a rate of 25% because inequities in the background studies may make the first test appear to be more accurate than the second. Although one might suppose that an overly inclusive approach to battery construction offsets such possibilities, one obviously cannot include everything. Additionally, as set forth in the materials on data integration, the inclusion of relatively weaker variables, even if they are valid, commonly has a negative influence on decision accuracy. As also follows from inflated study outcomes, error rates in clinical and forensic application can be considerably greater than research suggests, and the proportion of false-negative and false-positive errors can shift dramatically. As we will show, a marked increase in false-positive errors may be a common outcome. Surely it would be good policy in meta-analyses to separate results for studies that do and do not use comparable groups and determine if the findings vary.

We do not mean to paint a gloomy picture. Although we believe the EGP is an under-recognized and extremely important methodological problem, we also believe that methods can be developed to measure, account for, and attenuate or correct its influences and that this should be among the highest priorities for researchers in this area. At the end of this section, we suggest a number of possible research strategies and corrective approaches, and interested readers can also consult Ahern (2010) for further details about the EGP in general and potential strategies for addressing it.

The EGP stems from four basic sources which apply to a wide range of research in psychology (and likely other areas of "soft" science). First, as already described, there is a sensible desire to form groups with as few false members as possible. A second source relates to the nature of many entities and constructs in psychology that merit our attention and interest. These entities and constructs are often highly heterogeneous or show wide variation within classes. Examples include "executive functions," "attention," "aphasia," and, of course, "malingering." Such heterogeneity frequently results in part from limits in our classification systems and knowledge, but it is also intrinsic to many of the classes and constructs with which we have to deal.

A third source is the common lack of procedures that, in a sizeable percentage of cases, achieve definitive or near-definitive accuracy in determining who does and does not fall within the class of interest or whether a complex set of behaviors do or do not belong within the class. It is this difficulty or ambiguity that often motivates the researcher in the first place. As scientific knowledge advances, the percentage of individuals or occurrences that can be classified more definitively commonly increases, which redirects attention to the more ambiguous cases, creating an unsettling but imperfect paradox. We wish to learn how to classify the remaining ambiguous cases accurately, but in order to do so our research efforts are hampered by the very same problem we are setting out to address. To use a concrete, albeit inexact, analogy to illustrate the point, how could we study the nature and characteristics of trees if we often did not know how to identify trees in the first place? The dubious approach that may be commonly taken is to study the cases we do know how to identify in order to try to learn about the cases we do not know how to identify, which often produces pseudo-knowledge that nevertheless may fool us into thinking we are getting somewhere. We are better off realizing that the seeming paradox is incomplete, permitting means to attack the problem (most of which involve some form of bootstrapping, as we will describe).

Fourth, and related to the first three problems, the types of cases we do know how to identify are often extreme and unusually clean manifestations of the entity or construct under study and hence may apply minimally to the cases of greatest clinical interest and challenge. For example, when individuals perform below chance level on almost every test with a forced-choice format, accuracy in identifying malingering is likely to be very high. However, including these individuals in research groups in order to try to learn something about malingerers who are considerably more skilled and subtle may produce outcomes that are systematically misleading and do not improve but rather diminish accuracy, even to levels below that of a coin toss.

Figure 10 provides a schematic summary of the EGP and aspects of its interface with research and practice. For the sake of clarity, we start with the basic distinction between the presence and absence of malingering, and will later move on to the higher levels of complexity that are more typical in legal evaluations. Among all litigants for whom neuropsychological evaluation is performed, some are not malingering (M−) and some are malingering (M+). The certainty with which M− and M+ cases can be identified varies, and as before we have used the terminology D/ND (for definitive, near-definitive) and AMB (for ambiguous) to reflect surety of identification. In Fig. 10, however, rather than treating these designations as dichotomous

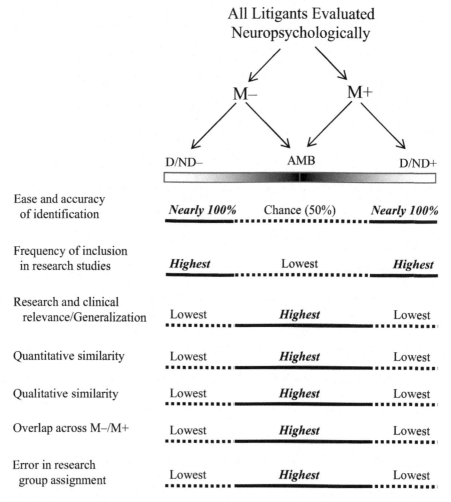

Fig. 10 Summary of extreme group problem (EGP) in relation to research and practice

categories, we have placed them on a continuum. The D/ND M– and M+ cases occupy the extremes, and as one moves toward the middle from either end the cases become more ambiguous, with the most ambiguous cases occupying the middle area. As we have emphasized, a major priority for research is reducing the percentage of remaining ambiguous cases. *Ease and accuracy of identification* represents another way of expressing standing on this continuum of definitiveness/ambiguity.

Examining the remaining entries and their relation to research priorities raises obvious concerns. Individuals who fall near the extremes of the continuum (e.g., definitive and near-definitive cases, subjects in simulation studies) have the highest *Frequency of inclusion in research studies* on malingering. However, the cases of greatest *Research and clinical relevance/Generalization* fall in the middle of the continuum. For reasons we have touched on and will further elaborate shortly, studies on extreme cases may not only generalize poorly to more ambiguous cases but may well lead to reliance on indicators that minimally enhance or even diminish accuracy. *Quantitative similarity* and *Qualitative similarity* reflect the potential for changes on these dimensions when one moves from more extreme to less extreme cases. For example, failure on certain test items that research suggests are indicative of malingering may instead be more highly associated with true injury. (These sorts of reversals are not nearly as unusual as they might seem, the literature on "scatter" and neuropsychological status providing multiple potential examples (see Faust et al., 2011).) *Overlap across M–/M+* also addresses the potential for qualitative shifts.

Error in research group assignment goes straight to the dilemma that ultimately creates extreme groups. When research groups are formed, all else being equal, error in group assignment is highly undesirable. For example, it would be exceedingly problematic if we drew research subjects from the very middle of the continuum, in which case about half of the subjects in the "malingering" group would be nonmalingerers and about half of those in the "control" group would be malingerers—we obviously would be pushing further and further into ignorance and error. We do not question whether erroneous group assignment should be a serious concern or whether, when it goes too far, it may not only inhibit progress but also lead us in the reverse direction (because much of what we thought we were learning would be wrong). However, minimizing error in group assignment should not necessarily trump all other considerations in research design, and if taken too far, as we believe too often happens in malingering research, it may greatly inhibit research progress. In part, whether we are going too far can be measured by examining the extent of the EGP. In many cases in science, using valid but fallible indicators for group assignment and then applying, to the extent possible, means to account for group impurity, is a crucial or even necessary step for achieving progress. Fallible group assignment is *not* a desirable end point, but it can be a necessary means for moving in the right direction.

Figure 11 illustrates the researcher's dilemma in malingering research. Put simply, in the usual circumstance, the purer the group the less relevant or helpful the research in addressing the most pressing current clinical needs (and the greater the likelihood the findings will be misleading). Across the sciences, such associations tend to hold to the extent the four factors or sources that create the EGP are present. In malingering research, at present, group purity almost always comes at the cost of selecting extreme cases. Thus, overprioritizing purity renders too much research of limited value or even potentially misleading for areas of current clinical need. It is essential to increase the level of clinical relevance without introducing too much error in classification, or to find means to compensate or account for it where feasible.

The potential for quantitative and qualitative shifts and resultant impact on error rates can be explained and illustrated through a series of figures. Staring with quantitative shifts, we turn to Fig. 12. To distinguish between malingerers and nonmalingerers in applied versus research settings, we will use the designation C for clinical and R for research. We know there can be overlap in these groups. For example, a

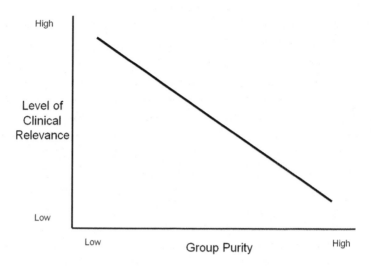

Fig. 11 Relationship between research group purity and degree of clinical relevance of research findings

researcher may cull presumed malingerers from applied settings, and the intent here is to first demarcate the totality of individuals in applied settings versus those that make up research groups.

The upper graph in Fig. 12 depicts ambiguous cases, those that tend to present the greatest diagnostic challenges and hence create the greatest research needs. In many such cases, there is a viable basis to suspect malingering. Of those suspected of malingering, some are malingering but others are not, and distinguishing between the two is not straightforward. We have previously referred to these subtler or less extreme cases with either the designation MS (suspected malingerers) or AMB (ambiguous cases), the latter of which appears in the current figure. In the top of Fig. 12, CM− (AMB) designates individuals in clinical or applied settings that are not malingering and CM+ (AMB) individuals who are malingering, with the AMB added to both groups to indicate that the cases are not obvious.

In the top half of Fig. 12, we have drawn hypothetical distributions that might apply to a modestly robust indicator, such as a score on a malingering subtest that achieves a .50 separation between the groups. Note that *both* groups have elevated averages relative to the mean of zero for the indicator, something which is often to be expected because individuals are suspected of malingering for a reason. Thus, it is not only the group that is *suspected of malingering and is* malingering that achieves elevated scores, but also the group that is *suspected of malingering but is not* malingering. What distinguishes the groups is not elevated scores per se but relative levels of elevation. In Fig. 12, the CM− group has a mean score of +1.00 SD and the CM+ group a mean of +1.50 SD. As one can see by consulting research on the MMPI-2, for example (see Greene, 2011), it is quite common for individuals with genuine disorders to score above the mean on malingering indices, one reason being that detection rests in part on overendorsement of items that have a true

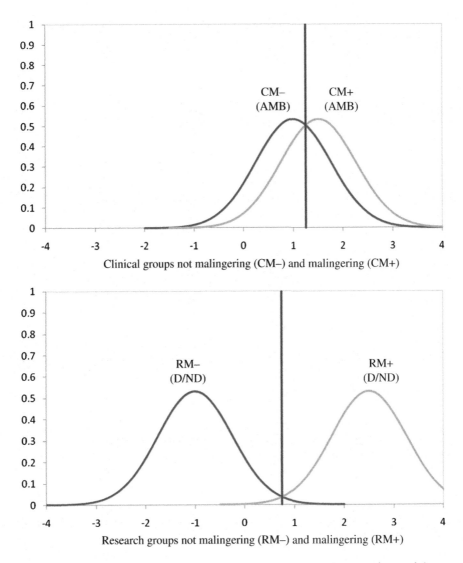

Fig. 12 Differences in score distributions for clinical (more ambiguous) cases and research (more definitively identified) groups

association with pathology. Consequently, in comparison to normal groups, scores are deviant, although usually only to a modest degree. Also, partly because so many effect sizes in malingering research are grossly inflated, one might think a figure like .50 is feeble or unfairly low. However, .50 reflects a fairly robust and helpful relationship, especially for an isolated indicator or score. With these means for the two groups, the optimal cut would likely fall at around 1.25 (although one might want to shift it to the left or right if false-positive or false-negative errors were a higher priority).

The bottom graph in Fig. 12 depicts distributions on the same indicator for research groups whose members have been identified definitively or near-definitively (D/ND) as malingering (RM+) or not (RM−). Based on having examined many studies on malingering detection, we would submit that the distributions we have drawn for these two groups are not rare. As one can see by referring back to Fig. 9, which was based on the Rogers et al. (2003) and Vickery et al. (2001) meta-analyses, between 22% and 32% of the outcomes exceeded effect sizes of 3.00. When one examines research across a range of malingering indicators, it is not difficult to find extraordinarily large effect sizes. Naturally enough, if authors point to indicators that yield the highest effects sizes as the most valuable ones, then practitioners will often be operating on the basis of distributions much like the ones that appear in the lower part of Fig. 12 (even though they are mainly an artifact of the EGP). We have not tried to represent the worst-case scenario or something even close to it, such as the third and fourth columns of effect sizes listed earlier (i.e., to save the reader from backtracking: 5.30, 5.47, 5.74, 6.53, 8.14, 10.24, 10.38, 13.66).

Compared to the CM+ group (the clinical malingerers) in the upper portion of Fig. 12, the RM+ group has shifted 1.00 SD to the right (from +1.50 SD to +2.50 SD). In comparison to the CM− group, the RM− group has shifted 2.00 SD to the left (from +1.00 SD to −1.0 SD). Each research group is more extreme than its corresponding clinical group, although the shifts are not symmetrical, with the CM− group shifting more than the CM+ group, hence changing the optimal cutting score from about +1.25 to about +.75 SD. Asymmetrical shifts are probably common, with the CM− group changing more than the CM+ group. The tendency toward asymmetrical shifts can be explained as follows. In clinical settings, we are starting with groups that are suspected of malingering (CM− and CM+), both of which usually obtain above average or elevated scores on malingering indicators. Consequently, in research settings, when we seek one group for which malingering is a near certainty (RM+) and another for which nonmalingering is a near certainty (RM−), we often need to move further from the clinical baseline in the latter instance because the standing of the CM− group is likely to fall in the abnormal range. The typical subject for whom there is no reason to suspect malingering is often "cleaner" than the typical clinical case or even control case, and thus the distance one must travel along the distribution of scores to reach something approaching definitely not malingering is often past the point of normality (relative to scores on the measure of interest).

The impact of these shifts, especially when asymmetrical, can be very deleterious. First, research studies will produce highly inflated accuracy rates or effect sizes, which is exactly what happens on many occasions. The worse the EGP, the better the method will look. Second, to the extent the magnitude of the EGP varies across studies examining different malingering indicators and tests, the greater the distortion in the relative efficacy of methods. We think there are strong reasons to assert that the EGP often exerts a far greater impact on study outcomes than the intrinsic properties of measures, and hence rank orderings of procedures are error prone, leading to practitioners often substituting weaker methods for stronger ones. Third, and perhaps most concerning, asymmetrical shifts distort optimal cutting scores. If the shifts are greater for the RM− group, which we think is the more common occurrence here, it will increase the false-positive rate, and if the shift is in the other direction it will increase the false-negative rate. One can see in Fig. 12 that the optimal cutting score has shifted .50 SD to the left, the result being that the CM− group mean now exceeds the cutting score by about .25 SD. As a consequence, *about 60% of those who are not malingering will be misidentified—the false-positive error rate now exceeds the outcome that would result by flipping a coin!* In a criminal context, should the shift go in the other direction, violent offenders feigning mental incompetence might be missed in a large percentage of cases. Although these graphs are hypothetical, the basic phenomena described here are real, and a magnitude of error that equals or exceeds that set forth in this example can be expected at times.

Thus far we have illustrated what we call quantitative shifts. Qualitative shifts can also occur and compound error. We do not wish to enter into pseudo-debates about qualitative and quantitative indicators because, as noted previously, almost any qualitative indicator can be quantified, rendering many arguments about relative merits moot. Suppose instead we make the distinction between continuous variables and dichotomous variables, the latter of which cover almost all the forms of "qualitative" data referred to in these debates. We would simply argue that all forms of data should be subject to formal study and testing when possible and judged on the basis of scientific merit rather than ideological positions. Surely at times, dichotomous distinctions can be of value (e.g., breathing or not, bizarre delusions present or absent, operable or inoperable tumor, performance that is or is not well below chance on multiple forced-choice methods). Various characteristics or red flags have been proposed as malingering indicators, a number of which can be conceptualized as dichotomous and which may well have value.

With common study designs, investigators recruit research group members they can identify definitively or almost definitively to try to learn how to identify clinical or forensic cases we do not know how to identify. This approach more or less guarantees some differences in the outset between the study subjects and the ultimate group to whom we wish to generalize the research (the AMB groups). If those in the AMB groups shared the characteristics of the individuals we can identify as D/ND malingerers and nonmalingerers, then they would not be AMB cases. Additionally, because of positive and negative manifold in psychology (good things are usually associated with other good things, and bad things with other bad things; see Meehl, 1990), ineffectual malingerers that are relatively easy to identify probably differ in more ways than the indicators used to identify them for purposes of the study (e.g., they may be less intelligent on average, more likely to present highly implausible symptoms, feign too broadly and grossly, have more difficulty keeping track of lies, or make less effort to prepare). Similarly, the control subjects, who are usually individuals for whom there is little or no reason to suspect malingering, likely also differ from their counterparts.

Figures 13 and 14 illustrate what we refer to as qualitative shifts and potential reversals. For purposes of illustration, we will designate our qualitative indicator as sign X. Perhaps it is recognition memory markedly below spontaneous recall, early

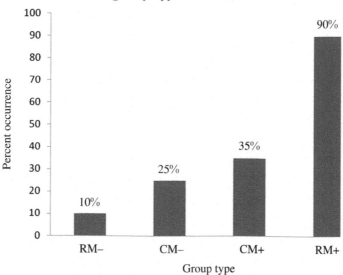

Fig. 13 Reduction in differential frequency from research to clinical groups

failures on easy test items, avoidance of eye contact, long response latencies, approximate answers, or some other such potentially differentiating feature. We may also have background studies (using extreme groups) that seem to support sign X. In any case, when selecting individuals for our current study the presence of sign X is considered an aid for identifying malingerers. If it presents along with certain other potential indicators (e.g., failure on forced-choice items), that individual is selected for the malingering group. When examining exclusionary criteria for the control group, the presence of more than one sign of malingering eliminates the individual from consideration. Given these selection criteria, few individuals in the nonmalingering group demonstrate sign X and most in the malingering group do demonstrate sign X. As one can see in Fig. 13, the RM− group demonstrates a frequency of 10% and in the RM+ group a frequency of 90%. If, as is sometimes done, the composition of each group is itself considered informative about the characteristics of malingering, then in rather circular fashion one might conclude that sign X is a strong differentiating sign, occurring nine times more often in malingerers than nonmalingerers. (This, unfortunately, is almost exactly the type of circular process used when depending on clinical experience to try to determine the characteristics of malingering.) Additionally, almost anything that correlated strongly with sign X, say, sign Y, might also show similar differential frequency.

Given the strategy of group formation, however, the relative frequencies of sign X or sign Y might be very different in applied settings. In Fig. 13, sign X is still valid for distinguishing the clinical groups (CM− and CM+) but not nearly as strong an

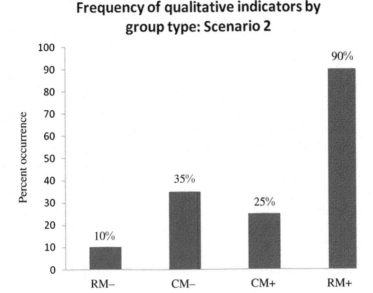

Fig. 14 Reversal in differential frequency for research to clinical groups

indicator as the research study suggests, and, depending on base rates and the availability of other indicators, a practitioner might be better off not using it at all. For example, if a strong alternative indicator is available, it will often conflict with sign X, and in the great majority of instances when one defers to sign X over the stronger indicator it will result in error.

Figure 14 illustrates what we refer to as reversal. Here, the relative frequency of the qualitative indicator is reversed among individuals in the applied setting; that is, the presence of the sign is in fact more common in the nonmalingerers than the malingerers. Lack of validity or reversal is not an outlandish outcome when extreme groups are selected because the characteristics of these groups and correlated features are unlikely to generalize to the AMB cases in applied settings. For example, gross failure on some malingering indicator may be common among research subjects but almost never observed among AMB cases. It is not hard to generate potential situations in which reversal might occur. For example, more severe cases of PTSD may be associated with higher rates of noncompliance. More severe brain injury cases may be associated with considerable response latencies; greater inconsistencies in performance due to such factors as easy fatigability, increased impulsivity, and attentional lapses; or certain elevations on personality tests that could be mistaken for overreporting or antisocial tendencies.

To summarize to this point, potential differences in amount and kind are often major obstacles to generalization from research studies to applied settings. They not only may distort or inflate accuracy rates, sometimes leading to gross overestimates and dangerously inflated confidence, but often do so unequally across studies and analyses of indicators, obscuring or reversing their relative standing. Furthermore, asymmetrical shifts in the extremity of malingering and control groups from research to clinical settings may alter cutting scores, markedly increase the frequency of false-negative or false-positive errors, and lead us to believe that qualitative indicators that are minimally effective or even reverse indicators of group status have considerable value. In many instances, all of this may be happening under our noses without our necessarily recognizing what is occurring. To those who take this to mean we are better off if we instead trust our clinical judgment and experience, it is highly likely that each and every one of the aforementioned problems will be no better and likely worse should those alternatives be selected. We also will not work our way out of these problems experientially, but require well-directed scientific efforts. Almost all of the considerable gains in malingering detection have ultimately been achieved through research, and there seems to be no compelling reason to think this situation will change. However, the distance remaining to be traveled in malingering detection may be a good deal further than is sometimes assumed.

It is sobering to think that we have set forth a simplified set of circumstances. Figure 15 (an elaboration on Fig. 5) displays relations between the EGP and joint presentations. For each of the four groups, the respective shaded areas of concern reflect overlap with other groups and hence ranges of outcomes that often create the greatest diagnostic difficulties. For example, if an individual who is not injured but is malingering obtains extremely poor results on forced-choice testing, the presence of malingering is likely to be recognized (although, arguably, a false identification of injury could still occur). The interested reader can turn back to the earlier section, "Mixed Presentations: Injured and Malingering," which covered the rationale for the positioning and widths of the shaded areas, and there is no need to reiterate those points here.

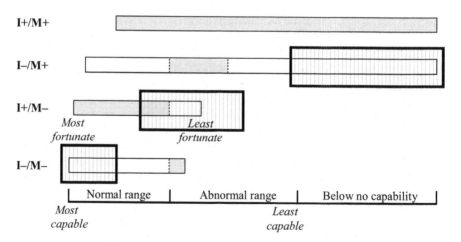

Fig. 15 Relation of areas of concern to research groups (patterned boxes)

The boundaries set forth in the boxes superimposed on certain sections of the entries for the I−/M+, the I+/M−, and the I−/M− groups identify typical compositions of research groups. For example, when the intended study group is malingerers (who presumably are not injured as well), researchers often focus on extreme cases to minimize error in group assignment; similarly, clean or extreme cases may be selected for a normal group. For injured groups, researchers often seek to identify individuals who clearly are injured and clearly are not malingering. The end result is that very little research focuses on AMB cases for which the diagnostic challenges are greatest; furthermore, due to potential quantitative and qualitative shifts, what is learned might not get us very far or may even be frankly misleading. Finally, the I+/M+ group contains no box identifying typical compositions in research studies because, despite the great importance of this category, there is almost no research on it. If the reader finds him- or herself getting a methodological stomachache at about this time, we can only say that all of the authors have shared the feeling. However, no one ever said that good science was easy, and we believe that these problems can be addressed productively through concentrated effort. A number of suggestions follow.

Possible Strategies for Addressing the EGP

It is sensible to be concerned about error in group assignment, but not to the point of generating research so encumbered by the EGP that it is of little or no value or even systematically misleading. Although minor or even modest problems in this area might not be so damning for exploratory projects in the context of discovery, it is a major shortcoming in the context of verification. Research on two basic fronts may assist in attacking the problem. First, recognition, measurement, and attempts at attenuation or correction are all worthy goals. Second, rather than learning to live with the problem or devising means to lessen its influence, we would be better off to avoid it in the first place. We will address both areas here, and more detailed discussion can be found in Ahern (2010), Bridges et al. (2009), and Faust et al. (2009b).

There are multiple ways to identify and measure the EGP. Examining the formation of research groups is one key. For example, cues to the presence and extent of the EGP include the number and breadth of inclusionary and exclusionary criteria and the percentage of potential subjects excluded from a study. Another tip-off is wildly fluctuating accuracy rates or effect sizes across studies on the same measure. One can examine whether "accuracy" seems to vary systematically with the extremity of groups, and how closely those groups resemble the cases of clinical interest. Large or outlandish effect sizes are strong indicators, as are implausible accuracy rates.

In some cases, accuracy rates exceed plausible levels given limits in the reliability of measures, this occurring because one is not studying a representative sample of cases but rather cases toward the extreme ends of distributions. Reliability figures reflect not only the intrinsic quality of tests but also the extremity of the groups studied. Thus, for example, depending on the metric used, an analysis of reliability based on the full distribution of cases can yield a lower result than examination of extreme cases drawn from both ends of the distribution. Suppose, for example, as is sometimes done, the consistency of classification is taken as an indicator of reliability. Here, if one mainly draws cases with very high or very low test scores, then even if there is considerable variation in results on retesting, decision consistency can still be very high. By way of analogy, if we are examining the consistency of first base umpires' decisions but primarily limit ourselves to cases in which the runner is either out or safe by a wide margin, then even if decision consistency is not very good on many calls and more typical situations, very high consistency rates may still be obtained. If a method with reliabilities in the .60s or .50s when used with broad samples generates accuracy rates in the 90% range in a separate study, there is a very good chance that the EGP is operating.

It is almost always worth checking within or across meta-analyses that compare the efficacy of different measures or indicators for the same diagnostic categories or outcomes. When study groups overlap entirely, the EGP is held constant, and this should often reduce or eliminate its confounding effects on the relative performance of measures. Of course, to the extent the EGP is present, accuracy rates may still be grossly inflated, cutting points may be shifted, and reductions or reversals of qualitative indicators may still occur. Nevertheless, barring interaction effects or certain forms of nonlinearity, the relative merits and rank ordering of methods should be preserved. If some studies have group overlap and some do not, one can compare outcomes across the overlapping and non-overlapping studies to look for trends. We would humbly suggest that journal editors keep this problem in mind and require that comparative analyses of methods separate the overlapping and non-overlapping studies and examine whether systematic differences result. Test A might beat test B when study groups overlap, but a meta-analysis may have pooled the overlapping and non-overlapping studies and altered the comparative outcome. It may be a mistake to think that the presence or absence of overlap is unlikely to be systematically related to the performance of the same indicator (e.g., the F scale on the MMPI-2). For example, better designed and well-funded studies may be more likely to include a broader range of indicators.

Probably the best solution to the EGP is to recruit representative samples. This is often a difficult undertaking for various reasons, in particular because one would need accurate methods to identify positive and negative cases across the range of possible (or at least relatively frequent) presentations, and it is the need for such knowledge that often drives the studies in the first place. If we had this knowledge we probably would not need to perform the study, and we are performing the study because we lack this very knowledge. Approaches that may assist in recruiting more representative samples (e.g., Group Membership by Chance) are discussed below.

In the meantime or as supplemental strategies, researchers may feel freer to recruit more relevant but less pure groups if approaches can be used to assess or adjust for error in group classification. One such approach is mixed group validation, also described below. For the remainder of this section, we wish to lay out what we have elsewhere labeled the *Definitive/Near Definitive Variation Rate* (DVR). We first described this method in Faust, Bridges, and Ahern (2009b), but it is possible we were not aware of precedents from which we unwittingly borrowed and hope we are not failing to properly credit the work of others.

As we have discussed, restricting studies to extreme cases is likely to yield misleading results. A fundamental factor impeding generalization is that the procedure used for forming research groups depends on characteristics (detectability) that set these participants apart from those that are not selected. However, it is the latter group—the group we presently cannot detect or have greater trouble detecting—that we are trying to determine how to detect more effectively. Group formation is thereby inevitably tied to a feature (detectability) that distinguishes the research subjects from the group we want to learn about, and that feature may also be associated with various other characteristics that separate these groups. The ultimate result is often lack of generalization to the group of greatest clinical interest or, even worse, "indicators" that are negatively associated with malingering (reversals).

The DVR strategy capitalizes on the occurrence of D/ND cases. Assume that across groups of malingerers (M+), the percentage that can be identified definitively or nearly definitively (D/ND M+) is fairly constant, and that the D/ND rate is also fairly constant for nonmalingerers (M−). Although the D/ND M+ rate and the D/ND M− rate each need to be fairly constant, the respective rates do not need to be consistent with one another. For example, it would not matter if the rate for the D/ND M+ cases is twice as high as the rate for the D/ND M− cases. Furthermore, when starting out, one does not even need to know what either of these rates might be, so long as there are strong reasons to assume they are both significantly above 0%, which is certainly the case. For purposes of illustration, we will assume a hypothetical D/ND rate of 40% for both the M+ and M− cases (leaving 60% from each group as ambiguous cases).

Assuming that 40% of malingerers can be identified definitively or nearly definitively, it follows that *if* we could randomly select, say, 1000 malingerers, then about 40%, or 400 subjects, would be classified as D/ND M+ cases. (We use the qualifier *if* because at present there is no method to identify such representative samples of malingerers.) Conversely, if we were able to randomly select a representative sample of 1000 individuals who were *not* malingering and evaluated each one, 0% (or close to 0%, given the potential for some error) would be classified as D/ND M+. We have also assumed that about 40% of nonmalingerers can be identified definitively or nearly definitively. Consequently, working from our hypothetical sample of 1000 malingerers, 0% (or close to 0%, given the potential for some error) would be classified as D/ND M− cases. Among the hypothetical sample of 1000 nonmalingerers, about 40%, or 400, would be classified as D/ND M− cases.

Although we are about to add one more set of hypothetical figures, we wish to emphasize that all of the figures set forth in this section are being used solely for illustrative purposes. Use of the DVR procedure also does not require, as noted, knowledge of the D/ND rates for malingering or nonmalingering groups, nor does one require knowledge of base rates for malingering. Furthermore, it is not necessary to identify representative groups of malingerers and nonmalingerers. Even evaluations for the occurrence of malingering and the separation of individuals into D/ND versus ambiguous cases do not need to achieve a high degree of accuracy. The more accurate the classifications the better, but the procedure should be able to tolerate even a moderately high error rate. The critical point for now is that the total number of D/ND M+ cases and D/ND M− cases should vary markedly (in this illustration from 400 to about 0) across the extremes, that is, depending on whether one is drawing from a sample with all malingerers versus a sample with no malingerers.

Again, working with a hypothetical figure, assume that the base rate for malingering among litigants seen for neuropsychological evaluation is 15%. Given this base rate, if one draws a random sample of 1000 such litigants, 150 individuals will be malingering and 850 will not be malingering. (We realize by dichotomizing the presence or absence of malingering we are simplifying matters and disregarding conjoint presentations, but again our major intent here is clarity, and the same principles should apply with more complex situations.) If the percentage of individuals who can be identified as D/ND M+ is a relative constant and falls at about 40%, as we have assumed for this illustration, then 40% of these 150 malingerers, or about 60, will be so identified. If the percentage of individuals that can be identified as D/ND M− is also about 40%, then about 340 of the 850 nonmalingerers will be so identified.

These potential outcomes can be summarized as follows, in each case assuming a sample size of 1000:

	D/ND M+	D/ND M−
Condition 1. An all malingering group yields:	400	0
Condition 2. An all nonmalingering group yields:	0	400
Condition 3. Random sampling yields:	60	340

These are the identical outcomes that would result were the first group formed by using a variable with perfect accuracy in identifying the presence and absence of malingering and only positive D/ND cases were selected; if the second group were formed using this same variable and only negative D/ND cases were selected; and if the third group were formed using a variable with no validity (and consequently was equivalent to random selection). We will use the term *comparison ratio* to refer to the result produced by a variable with no validity.

Suppose now we were able to draw a random sample of litigants undergoing neuropsychological evaluation, thereby providing the needed comparison ratio for research with this group. Based on background knowledge, we have estimated the base rate for malingering in our sample as modest to relatively low (e.g., 15%). Hence, we have a good idea about outcome if we identify all of the D/ND M+ and D/ND M− cases in our sample: we will have a considerably lower number of M+ as opposed to M− cases, with a ratio approximating the one that appears under Condition 3 above, which is about 60:340, or about 1:6 (rounding off to the nearest whole number). As noted, this is the same ratio expected if a variable had no validity, which provides the foundation for its use as the comparison ratio. We need not know this ratio in advance; we derive it through random sampling of the overall group of interest, followed by evaluating the sample and identifying D/ND M+ and D/ND M− cases.

In contrast to a variable that has no capacity to differentiate between group members, as validity increases, the comparison ratio will shift accordingly. Consider Condition 1, which illustrates the hypothetical result expected with a variable at the far end of the spectrum, or one with perfect accuracy in identifying the presence and absence of malingering. Here if we select the first 1000 *positive* cases, evaluate these individuals, and identify D/ND M+ and D/ND M− cases, the obtained ratio should be about 400:0, which is far different than the comparison ratio of 1:6! If this same variable is used to select the first 1000 *negative* cases, the obtained ratio should be about 0:400, again an extreme departure.

Although we would almost never anticipate such huge shifts, it does follow that the more valid a variable for separating group membership, the larger the shift. Therefore, it would seem feasible to measure a variable's validity and also to place it along an ordinal scale that reflects relative level of validity: the greater the shift, the higher its standing on the scale. One could also examine the impact of combining variables, such as the extent to which adding a new variable yields incremental validity.

The potential value of the DVR method is that it does not require knowledge of base rates or knowledge of whether individuals are or are not malingering for the group studied as a whole, and it likely can tolerate at least moderate departures from representative sampling. We realize we have only presented the broad outlines of this strategy, it is in an early stage of development, and considerable further refinement is needed. A number of practical obstacles would also need to be addressed. We would not expect such research to be undemanding but do believe that the DVR method is feasible. Given the scope and importance of malingering assessment, the effort and resources that would be needed to appropriately test and develop this method seem to be justified.

5.3   Lack of Representative Samples

Identifying representative samples of malingerers and nonmalingerers (and mixed presentations of malingering conjoined with disorder) would obviously be of great benefit. Representative samples are crucial for determining which features are valid predictors and differentiate among groups, appraising generalization of signs and indicators, and deriving accurate base rates. Unfortunately, researchers are often faced with one of two problematic situations. In one they have recruited a group whose members are known to be malingering with near certainty, but one whose composition is almost surely nonrepresentative of malingerers as a whole, especially the cases we currently have difficulty detecting and for which help is most needed. This is a variation of the EGP discussed above. In the other circumstance, a group has been identified that is known to be relevant, but within that group one does not know in many cases who is and is not malingering. The latter circumstance almost always holds in contrasting group designs. Thus, we may be able to obtain a group representative of those applying for disability, but we do not know who may be malingering or to what degree, except perhaps for those who produce extreme outcomes and hence are not the cases we are trying to learn how to detect more effectively. The problem of determining the status of group members has limited the utility of contrasting group designs, although we believe there may be ways to augment these designs to increase their effectiveness (see below).

The seeming paradox is that one would need to know how to identify malingerers before recruiting representative samples, at which point one would not need to do the studies. The absence of representative samples, or rather the inability to determine whether samples are representative, greatly hinders efforts to identify and evaluate potential malingering indicators. Under such conditions, it is very easy to inadvertently adopt signs that are ineffectual or, even worse, increase the number of misidentifications.

Situational variables may also separate research subjects and settings from litigants in applied situations. Many malingerers, especially in brain damage cases, have experienced an injurious or potentially injurious event. Thus, for example, a researcher might try to recruit subjects who were in car accidents and seen in emergency rooms but did not suffer head injuries. Some malingerers have been exposed to models or mentors (e.g., a relative who has been injured or someone who has malingered successfully, such as a fellow prisoner). Many malingerers have met with attorneys prior to undergoing examinations, and a sincere attorney may provide inadvertent cues through leading questions about head injury, or may warn the client about malingering detection methods an independent examiner might use. Many malingerers have also been subjected to multiple medical examinations, including those in which feedback or "education" about injury is provided. For example, a neuropsychologist who discusses results with examinees may provide detailed information about head injury or even about her reasons for questioning the examinee's cooperation. If the attorney is unhappy with initial assessment results, a new examination might be sought and the prior examination not disclosed, with the plaintiff now far better forearmed to influence outcomes in a desired direction.

We would like to propose an approach that we think offers promise for obtaining more representative groups of real-world malingerers. We label this the *Group Membership by Chance* (GMC) strategy, and we believe it can be applied to a range of situations in the social sciences when conventional methods of random selection are problematic either because of ethical constraints (e.g., head injury studies) or because means for identifying individuals with the condition in question are weak or lack adequate validation. In usual circumstances, in order to obtain representative samples, one selects randomly from a known population. Thus, were it feasible, one would randomly sample the population of malingerers and then compare that group with other groups the clinician needs to distinguish. Unfortunately, it is not currently feasible to do so and we are generally limited to samples that are almost surely not representative—and very possibly systematically misrepresentative—of malingerers as a whole. The more basic problem is the absence of a method for evaluating just how representative that subgroup might be. Without such a method, even if one happens to obtain a representative group, one cannot determine that this good bit of fortune has occurred, and hence it really does no good.

Some malingerers are caught primarily because they are ineffectual malingerers. Others are caught primarily because they are unlucky. Take the following case in which one of the authors consulted. One of the professional staff, who had left the treatment setting at an unscheduled hour as a result of an unexpected personal circumstance, just happened to observe a patient, who momentarily let down his guard once he was blocks away from the hospital, exactly at the moment he engaged in an activity he absolutely should not have been able to do. Or in another circumstance, a plaintiff may have just happened to run into an unusually skilled and determined detective who caught him acting normally, whereas seven other malingering coworkers happen to have been assigned to more mediocre sleuths.

In the idealized instance, an individual who is caught entirely as a result of bad luck is directly parallel to a malingerer drawn randomly from the pool of malingerers, that is, she represents in essence an instance of random selection. If one can identify enough such individuals, one should be able to comprise a group that is likely to be representative of malingerers as a whole, or at least a good approximation. This allows not only for analysis of that GMC group, but also for checks on the representativeness of groups formed in other ways (e.g., malingerers identified by other means or cases compiled via contrasting group methods). It might also be possible to estimate the relative purity or base rates for malingering in contrasting groups, which offers major benefits, especially when studying generalization of measures across applied settings. For example, using methods designed by Dawes and Meehl (1966), and further advanced by such researchers as Jewsbury and Bowden (2014), if one can dsetermine the relative impurity of validation groups, one can then adjust for cases of false inclusion (i.e., the mixture of properly and improperly included individuals). The DVR method described earlier would also benefit from informed estimations about the mix of group members.

There are a number of questions and issues one might raise about such an approach, some of which can be touched on here (see also Faust, 1997). One question involves the methods used for determining the level of chance in identification. We think that this is not too difficult a methodological problem because: (a) the method does not require perfect indicators (one does not have to be particularly concerned about some impurity), (b) rational analysis should provide reasonable accuracy in estimating the contribution of chance, (c) failures of inclusion (false-negative errors) do not have distorting influences (one can be conservative if need be without worrying too much about consequential problems with representativeness), (d) the approach described here is an initial approximation to addressing what has been a longstanding and very difficult problem and can be refined over time, and (e) a variety of checks can be built into the procedure. For example, a series of risky predictions can be made that should hold if the method works.

A second problem is not conceptual or methodological but practical. How could one possibly find enough caught-by-chance subjects? It is probably unnecessary to limit the method to pure cases because if the level of chance can be estimated even approximately and accounted for, more lenient inclusionary criteria would probably be workable. Nevertheless, data pooling would seem essential. On a national level, there are surely many such cases. The question is how to garner them. This is one of various domains of malingering research in which efforts would be helped greatly if more funding were available to researchers. Given the presumed cost of fraud attributable to malingering, these might be dollars well invested. Alternatively or additionally, if large collaborating networks of neuropsychologists could be created, it could greatly facilitate this and other important data gathering initiatives.

5.4   Base Rates: Some Research Priorities

The value and utility of base rate information have already been described. In a range of situations, base rates are among the most useful, or the single most useful, diagnostic indicator or sign. Additionally, knowledge of base rates is often critical in determining the potential utility of test results or other assessment methods. Shifts in base rates alter ratios between true-positive and false-positive, and true-negative and false-negative identifications. Base rate information is needed to determine whether we should use signs at all, the accuracy that signs achieve, and whether and how we should adjust cutting scores. As was described above, professionals often seem to underweight base rates or have problems applying them properly, which can be viewed as a high-priority item for education and training programs given the benefits accrued from better practices. Fortunately, an increasing number of publications in neuropsychology that address diagnostic practices in general or malingering more specifically, as well as professional manuals, touch on the importance and application of base rates. On occasion these discussions arguably conflict with sound advice by instructing individuals to formulate and apply composite base rates for practice settings, by underemphasizing the limited value of global base rates, and perhaps by overstating the surety of current base rate information (see the earlier discussion, "*Recognizing flawed advice about the use of base rates*"). An even more fundamental problem is that articles or manuals may offer base rate estimates that vary widely and one generally does not know which estimate is most accurate or applicable in the setting of interest. Alternatively, global estimates may be provided, which are often of little value.

The problem with global estimates is not only their occasional wide variance but the limited value of such information, in and of itself. First, these global estimates are mainly guesses, and whether or not practitioners, for example, show some convergence in estimates, this is a soft evidentiary basis for determining accuracy. Second, the frequencies depend on a range of assumptions that may contain arbitrary elements, rest on insufficient knowledge, or do not address essential considerations. For example, frequencies will depend on where thresholds are set. If we equate almost any form of exaggeration with malingering, we are likely to obtain extraordinarily high rates, but if we set more stringent standards rates will likely decline sharply. This is a little like deciding the threshold for identifying friendliness and then claiming a certain resultant base rate is accurate. Third, almost none of the background studies include the conjoint category of malingering and injured, which, as we have described, can change obtained base rates and accuracy rates dramatically. A certain percentage of individuals who are malingering or exaggerating are also injured, and in some situations in which that frequency might be high, reporting a base rate for malingering or for genuine injury as if they were exclusive classes may be decidedly misleading. Fourth, and perhaps most importantly, when base rates for a condition vary widely across individuals, settings, and circumstances, which is almost surely the case here, global base rates are often of little utility. Such global base rates may minimally increase diagnostic and predictive accuracy, and in some cases may make no positive contribution or even diminish success.

We return here to the same type of paradox we encounter when attempting to determine how to best measure malingering—we need to know more than we know if we are to find out what we need to know. We need base rate information to appraise the accuracy of our diagnostic methods, and yet to determine base rates we need accurate measures of malingering. Nevertheless, it is commonplace in science to face such problems and yet to gradually evolve ways to overcome them, a process that is well underway in research on malingering detection.

Recognizing that global base rates are of minimal value, a key research priority is to determine how base rates vary across circumstances so that one can perform the type of reference group refinement described previously. The aim is to identify the base rate for the narrowest applicable group, with narrowness defined here by dimensions that: (a) alter the base rates and (b) are relevant to the individual under consideration. An obvious and important start is the presence or absence of financial incentive to malinger (e.g., involvement in legal proceedings), which, not surprisingly, seems to have a considerable impact on base rates (see Binder & Rohling, 1996; Frederick & Bowden, 2009; Reynolds, 1998). The larger the impact of variables, the less the remaining variance in base rates for which we need to account. Although one might think that a large number of factors are required, with these sorts of multivariate problems often a relatively small number of variables (perhaps three to five) are needed to reach or approach the ceiling in efficacy.

A number of investigatory strategies may assist in acquiring further base rate information and in identifying features that allow for determining differential frequencies among narrower groups. As already described, strategies for forming representative groups, such as the GMC method, may prove helpful. Meehl's previously described taxometric methods also provide a potential means for estimating base rates (see Meehl, 1995, 1999, 2001, 2004, 2006; Waller & Meehl, 1998). The DVR method also may help in base rate studies. For example, in some circumstances, the percentage of D/ND cases within a sample may provide a strong cue for overall malingering rates within that sample (see further below).

A variation of a contrasting group design should assist in estimating base rates across situations and groups, with its utility enhanced if combined with the DVR method. One could develop a series of contrasting groups, each with likely differences in level of effort. It would be helpful to add groups with positive incentives to perform well, such as individuals applying for financial assistance for educational or vocational funding or individuals applying for employment. Other circumstances with positive incentives might include custody evaluations, certain types of competency exams in which individuals want to perform well (e.g., competency to control one's finances or execute a will), and psychometric examinations that are part of appraisals for resumption of driving privileges or return to sports activities.

Some of these positive-incentive groups are likely to have malingering or poor effort rates that approach 0%, whereas the groups with the highest incentives to perform poorly may have rates that equal or exceed 50%. If, for example, one can determine or approximate the percentage of malingering cases that can be detected among all those who are malingering, and especially if this rate is reasonably constant (or at least predictable) across the groups, this should provide useful information about base rates.

For the sake of illustration, suppose about 25% of the cases can be detected with certainty or near certainty and that this rate of detection is relatively constant across the groups. One can then use the 25% figure to extrapolate the base rate for malingering within the various groups. For example, suppose that in a group of 100 with a very high incentive to malinger, 15 D/ND identifications are made. Assuming that 25%, or one in four individuals, who are malingering can be identified definitely or nearly definitively, the estimated bare rate for malingering in the group is 4 × 15, or 60 individuals, resulting in an estimated base rate of 60%. Of course, additional studies with similar groups would be needed to examine consistency in outcomes and develop firmer estimates of base rates. Across groups with differing levels of incentive to malinger, if the percentage of D/ND cases is a relative constant, then the same method of extrapolation can be used to estimate their respective base rates. If, instead, the percentage of D/ND cases varies across the groups, which is not unlikely, estimating base rates becomes more difficult, but various approaches can be used, such as the DVR method, to approximate percentages of D/ND cases and move forward from there.

Study of performance characteristics within and across groups might help in identifying valid and differentiating diagnostic signs and indicators and in identifying features that alter base rates and help in narrowing groups. If certain features appear much more commonly among the high frequency groups and show a steady rise in frequency as incentives or malingering rates increase, they are promising indicators or potential factors that alter base rates. A variety of approaches would likely be needed to advance or verify results, and in such bootstrapping operations one especially looks for convergence or consistency among different indicators as a key method of validation (see Meehl, 1995). For example, it would be very interesting to examine whether potential indicators identified through such contrasting group designs were replicated in simulation studies. (In some circumstances, rather than starting with simulation studies and checking generalization to other circumstances, one could cross-check other research findings by subsequently performing simulations.)

Apart from contrasting group designs, there is at least one way researchers should be able to determine the lower limits of base rates. If one applies a measure with a very high true-positive rate, or measures on which positive results offer something close to *prima facie* evidence of malingering (at least on that task), then the obtained rate of positive identifications should provide a good estimate of minimum frequencies. For example, suppose performances that are well below chance on a forced-choice procedure could be taken as strong evidence for malingering. If this method was applied, say, to a group of disability applicants, the frequency of positive results should provide a minimal estimate of malingering rates. Of course, the true base rate might be substantially higher, but we would at least have a good approximation of the lower limit, and anything that allows us to start narrowing ranges is helpful. In many circumstances, even obtaining very rough estimates of upper and lower boundaries can give us clear pragmatic guidance. For example, some signs would prove effective, and some ineffective, anywhere within the range. Application of the strategy suggested here would probably uncover some situations in which our minimal estimates are erroneous, permitting us to sharpen our knowledge of base rates.

We might be able to do a good deal better in estimating minimal frequencies if we use multiple assessment devices or approaches with high true-positive rates, taking positive results of any of these measures as evidence of malingering. For example, we might look for positive results on symptom validity testing, direct evidence that the individual can perform normally in areas in which disability is claimed (e.g., video recordings), and confessions. Some individuals might confess at the time of evaluation, and others might confess if granted absolute assurances about immunity or after a nonreversible determination is reached. When formulating estimates on this basis, the conjunctive false-positive error rate of the measures would need to be taken into account. The major advantage of such a combined approach is reduction in the false-negative rate because, at present, approaches that appear to have high true-positive rates also seem to have high false-negative rates. We do not imagine that these types of combined approaches would be easy to pursue; but the effort would seem to be justified by the enormous benefits we gain if we are able to formulate reasonable estimates of the base rates. One would also think that the value of such knowledge could lead to favorable funding decisions.

5.5 Transparency

Most methods of malingering detection fall into one of four groups: they look for instances in which individuals perform (a) less well than they can, (b) less well than they should, or (c) differently than they ought to; or they (d) capitalize on stereotypic misconceptions about pathology (the last two categories could arguably be combined). These various approaches usually either depend on examinees holding some type of faulty belief, or they attempt to induce some false assumption. Attempts to induce false beliefs or assumptions vary in sophistication, power, and ease of detection (by the examinee). In some cases, an examinee is told that a test that is practically shouting out, "Try me, I'm easy," is really difficult, and then must perform miserably on the measure to be identified as a possible malingerer. In contrast, the MMPI-2 F scale depends on false stereotypes about disorder, which may be shared by laypersons and mental health professionals alike (e.g., see Gough, 1954). Simple attempts to educate oneself about disorder might not help. Rather, one needs to find out how the F scale operates and how to identify F scale items, and one then needs to endorse enough of those items to achieve an appropriate elevation but not so many items that one is caught. For many methods of malingering detection, should the instructions or test stimuli fail to create misbelief or if examinees discern the simple, one dimensional detection strategy, there is a good chance the procedure can be beaten (for what appears to be a striking exemplar, see Kovach & Faust, in preparation). And if the clinician interprets anything short of clearly malingered performance on one or a few such measures as presumptive evidence of good effort, the examinee is likely to beat the clinician as well. Many of our methods are much too transparent and are likely to lose much of the effectiveness they might have as word about how they work circulates.

It would be prudent to assume that the underlying design of a malingering detection method will be discovered and circulated over time. The question is how to extend the time period before they lose their effectiveness or to make them much more difficult to beat even if their underlying design is known. Given such realities as the exceptional motivation of some malingerers, the public nature of legal proceedings, the wide latitude given cross-examiners in challenging the underlying bases of conclusions, and the omnipresent internet, it is unrealistic to believe that trade secrets will not leak out.

We can think of various means to counter transparency, and undoubtedly others can expand or improve on the ideas provided here. First, problems with the transparency of forced-choice methods would likely be reduced immediately by increasing the number of foils. Further gains would be realized by varying the number of foils across items and randomizing the order in which items with varying numbers of foils appear. For example, suppose one had items with two to four foils. Suppose that each of these items required the individual to identify a previously presented word on a memory test. Further suppose that the order of the two-, three-, and four-foil items was randomized, such that one did not complete the items with any particular number of foils in a group. The task of producing plausible rates of successes and failures when trying to portray a serious memory disorder would seem to be immensely more difficult under such conditions than those in which, for example, the individual only needs to aim for a certain failure rate. This and other approaches can capitalize on limits in human cognition, such as restrictions in the ability to track multiple dimensions of a problem simultaneously.

In a related vein, we might also take advantage of limits in human memory. For example, if inconsistency in presentation helps to differentiate between malingerers and the genuinely disordered, we can create circumstances in which fakers likely must resort to making up answers as they go along and will probably have extreme difficulty reproducing their results at a later time. Suppose we compile a large number of items with low face validity that call for fairly rapid responses and have reasonable stability among honest reporters. A malingerer who does not know how she should answer but is trying to alter her presentation will most likely fall into an arbitrary pattern of responding that is very difficult to repeat on a subsequent occasion given normal limits in recall. There are many other ways one could attempt to design procedures that require extraordinary or near-impossible memory feats if one is to produce plausible performances over time.

Current attempts to create mental sets about item difficulty might be checked directly against research participants' perceptions. For example, how hard does an item seem at first blush and to what extent do suggestions about item difficulty alter perceptions (especially among those warned that the examiner may sometimes mislead them)? If we are going to pursue such approaches, we might try to expand and refine our methods for creating misperceptions. Indirect verbal suggestion might sometimes be as or more effective than direct suggestion (e.g., telling someone that they will get five chances at materials versus telling them something is hard). Also, there would seem to be ways to alter perceptual impressions of difficulty without really changing objective difficulty, or in fact changing it in the opposing direction. For example, various perceptual illusions might be exploited to create misimpressions.

Other approaches might include shifting item pools and interspersing items that measure effort with items that measure ability. In the first instance, rather than having one set of items, if there were numerous parallel items that could be used in varying combinations, it would probably make identification of the test more difficult and extend the half-life of methods. With interspersed items (which also might be combined with the first approach), one would have to be careful not to contaminate standard measures. Thus, it might be preferable to embed ability and effort items together in the development stage if, for example, one were simultaneously developing a new measure of immediate visual memory and ways of measuring cooperation on the measure. Although potentially complex, one major advantage is that in cases of poor performance, one would be able to simultaneously evaluate effort. Additionally, one could develop parallel forms with separate norms that exclude effort items in situations in which the appraisal of malingering is a low priority and one does not want to lengthen measures unnecessarily.

If and when baseline neuropsychological data become more widely available, formal approaches that calculate fit with expectations for preserved and diminished functions relative to the injury in question as opposed to inadequate effort might gain greater effectiveness and be relatively difficult to feign effectively. In the meantime, inter- and intra-individual variability and overreliance on subjective appraisal greatly curtail the efficacy of such approaches. In fact, they may be as much or more a guessing game for the neuropsychologist as the examinee, and the potential for error is a serious concern.

We may also want to look at methods that start with subjective ratings of item difficulty, probing for misimpressions. We might eventually be able to develop a fairly large set of items or be able to alter dimensions on the spot to examine their influence on impressions. Thus, rather than hoping or guessing that a misimpression has been created, one would wait to receive some confirmation that it has occurred before proceeding with administration of items. We expect that in the future, much of neuropsychological and effort testing will use adaptive formats that make these sorts of procedures more readily achievable and routine.

With data pooling, it would be of interest to trace positive and negative rates on tests over time to provide a barometer of obsolescence. For example, if a measure that previously demonstrated, say, a 15% rate of positive results gradually showed a drop in comparable settings and circumstances, it might suggest that knowledge about how to beat the measure is becoming increasingly well known. More generally, when developing measures for assessing effort, examining transparency and vulnerability to knowledge of design could be considered essential and not something to pursue only after tests are published. These studies can include providing examinees with high-quality information about the measure's detection strategies. Additionally, sequential testing might be conducted, in the first instance without information about detection strategies and then after feedback is provided about performance or results, as might be the case in legal settings when individuals are examined on multiple occasions by the same or different neuropsychologists. There is little doubt that in many instances an individual who achieves results suggestive of poor effort is given some type of feedback about the outcome and is retested at a later date with the same or similar measures.

We are not suggesting that researchers abandon attempts to create measures that tap into false stereotypes. This approach has a long history of success, at least with the MMPI and MMPI-2, and we certainly should not demand that malingering detection devices catch everyone. Many individuals who malinger will not invest the time and effort needed to learn what they should do to effectively portray disorder, others will have difficulty mastering the needed knowledge and strategies, and initial evaluations may be performed before someone has a chance to become educated about the procedures. Additionally, methods that tap commonly held but false stereotypes may show limited redundancy with other approaches, which, as noted, increases their potential utility when combined with other predictors. Furthermore, if methods and approaches are consistently updated as knowledge advances, it may be possible to stay a step ahead of many malingerers. For these reasons, efforts to extend this type of approach to structured and semistructured interview techniques and questionnaires that are specifically targeted at neuropsychological and related disorders seem very much worthwhile, as well as continuing efforts to study lay perceptions of head injury and other neurological disorders (e.g., Wong et al., 1994). Such research can help in identifying candidate items for these types of malingering detection approaches.

5.6   Data Combination and Incremental Validity

As more malingering detection approaches are becoming available, showing that a single measure has discriminating power under one or another condition is minimally informative. Often, we will already have other measures that have passed the same hurdle, and one really needs to know how the new measure compares with other available methods and whether it makes a unique contribution to predictive accuracy. There is limited utility in identifying or developing indicators that are redundant with previously available methods. A study limited to showing that a new variable has discriminating power is usually of negligible help because we cannot evaluate whether that variable will have a negative, positive, or neutral effect on predictive accuracy when combined with other variables.

Rather, we should be trying to uncover variables that are likely to contribute unique predictive variance. It would be very beneficial if far greater effort was made to assess incremental validity, that is, any improvement gained by adding a new predictor to the best predictors that are already available. Given the inordinate demands that can be placed on subjective judgment, including the need to separate predictive and nonpredictive variables, gauge the strength of association between predictors and criterion, determine level of redundancy among predictors, and examine multiple possible ways of combining variables, it becomes imperative to have formal methods of data combination, and particularly actuarial or statistical procedures. The development of the most effective decision methods, by its nature, requires study of incremental validity.

Some investigators have examined multiple variables and their combined effects, which is a start; but too often these studies do not do much more than add to the innumerable demonstrations of a matter that is not at issue, that is, that the statistical combination of multiple valid predictors will usually outperform a single valid predictor. What these studies do not examine is the effect of combining new predictors with the best available predictors.

We cannot, however, perform all possible comparisons among measures and across conditions and variations of malingering. Blind empiricism is inefficient and usually ineffective in the long run. Rather, scientific efforts typically should be guided by principles, informed advice, and generalizations that usually hold. For example, it is completely impractical to test every conceivable comparison, and scientific and clinical practice often occur under conditions of uncertainty, in which there is no sure road. In such situations, however, one operating from well-founded guesses and principles has a huge advantage over someone operating blindly. Take the methodological guide: "A method shown to make fine discriminations should do even better making more gross distinctions." There are times this generalization is flat-out wrong (as might occur, for example, when the situation changes qualitatively), but we usually do not know this in advance, and rather we are trying to resolve a question under ambiguous conditions. In attempting to do so, our odds of being correct are much greater if we follow this generalization than if we guess randomly, and correct guesses can greatly enhance the productivity of our scientific efforts. When designing studies, we should especially keep in mind the advantages gained by pooling nonredundant measures.

There has been increased attention directed to combining measures and indicators in recent years (e.g., Bain et al., 2019; Bashem et al., 2014; Berthelson et al., 2013; Bilder et al., 2014; Davis & Millis, 2014; Erdodi, 2019; Erdodi & Abeare, 2019; Larrabee, 2014), although not a high volume of work. Studying incremental validity in the assessment of effort and malingering will require substantial effort and study given the complexities involved, such as the potential need to adjust combinations based on the disorders under consideration, individual differences (e.g., level of baseline functioning), and most probably a number of sociocultural factors. Some research has suggested that a certain proportion of abnormal results on measures of effort translate into certain percentages or ranges of likelihood, including in some cases a very high probability that effort is suboptimal. However, such results are often highly dependent on a series of conditionals that frequently shift across circumstance, application, and the specific measures used.

We have serious concerns that some of these higher figures for the likelihood of malingering overestimate probabilities by a significant margin and can cause considerable harm, as those conducting studies may well have pointed out themselves. Among the various reasons for such cautions, two seem especially worth emphasizing. One is the extreme group problem (EGP), which as noted often produces markedly inflated accuracy rates in comparison to rates obtained in clinical application. The other concern is that many malingering studies validate measures by establishing correlation or high association with other effort measures, practices that are likely to increase redundancy across the combination of measures practitioners may select. Level of incremental validity is optimized by selecting measures with the dual qualities of validity and relative independence from one another, and thus research emphasizing associations between measures routinely produces outcomes in which the measures that look best are redundant or highly redundant with one another. Consequently, when selecting what appear to be the best measures, the combinations that are picked may be considerably more redundant than desirable. In turn, exceptional rates of accuracy obtained in studies using less redundant measures and receiving a substantial, artificial boost from the EGP (likely inadvertently), may well yield accuracy rates far above those obtained in typical clinical and forensic practices.

Speaking more broadly about combining measures for assessing effort, Bilder et al. (2014, pp. 1220–1221) described a series of concerns that seem worth emphasizing. As they stated:

1. "We lack adequate theoretical, mathematical, or statistical models of PVT failure across multiple tests, so we need to rely on empirical data.
2. The empirical data show a clear impact of number of PVTs administered [relative to false positive rates].
3. The empirical data show a clear impact of patient factors, including general ability.
4. The existing empirical study designs must be examined carefully before applying specific rules to an individual case.
5. Empirical demonstrations should be evaluated carefully for redundancy between criteria for case selection and the methods for calculating false positive rates."

6   Caveats and Final Comments

6.1   Proposed Criteria for Malingering Detection

Various criteria for identifying malingering have been proposed, which can facilitate research and communication within the field. However, these proposals are clearly experimental, and there are strong grounds to question whether they should be used at present in legal cases. Those proposing criteria are often open and explicit about their tentative standing. Should experts nonetheless depend on such criteria, reading developers' cautionary passages may help establish their limits.

To an extent that may not be recognized, definitions or criteria follow from scientific knowledge and advance rather than the reverse. A questionable set of criteria based on insufficient knowledge can lead to nonproductive research efforts and misleading results. As an imperfect analogy but one that is illustrative, suppose we wished to learn about whales and prematurely defined them as animals that live in the sea, draw air from water, are all carnivorous, and are always over 50 feet long. Given such criteria, how much would we have learned, for example, about Belugas?

Similarly, operational definitions often do nothing to resolve critical conceptual issues, create a false sense of scientific resolution, and were abandoned by almost all philosophers of science decades ago (and nearly so by Bridgman (1927) at the end of his famous—or infamous—book in which he introduced the flawed concept). If malingering is what a malingering test measures, then that is what it had better do or the "definition" is erroneous. (However, repudiation of operational definitions should not be confused with the potential advantages of clear and explicit definitions, which is another matter.) Furthermore, as malingering is a hypothetical construct or latent entity, it follows that it cannot be reduced to a set of observations or observables because inference is always required. Thus, as the philosopher puts it, surplus meaning is involved, which should not be equated with a scientific sin.

6.2 Labeling

Labels assigned to results on malingering tests are sometimes highly misleading. Some tests adopt a very stringent threshold for identifying malingering, such as a probability of at least 90%. At times, even if the likelihood approaches this level but falls just short of it, the designated description or the expert's summary comment might be something like "within normal limits," or even "indicative of good effort." When a clinician indicates, for example, that an outcome is "unremarkable" or "confirms adequate effort," jurors probably would have no idea that chances might approach 9 out of 10 that effort on the test was poor or insufficient (and that a rather extreme standard was being used for the identification of malingering). Some experts describe almost any result that does not strongly indicate poor effort as demonstrating a satisfactory or high level of effort, which treats the matter as all or none and disregards degrees between these extremes. Similarly, defense experts who describe effort as inadequate or poor may not communicate how close the call was, or perhaps that the evidence was inconsistent. For example, they may emphasize one questionable result and underweight a number of other scores that fell within expected levels for the injury in question.

Descriptive or labeling practices should serve to provide accurate information and avoid misimpressions. Labeling practices often originate from the meritorious desire to avoid false-positive identification of someone as malingering (see further below), but to the degree labels create confusion in either direction, the trier of fact may well form inaccurate impressions. In general, it might be better to report both the probabilities and one's conclusions, instead of merely classifying the results one way or the other or providing an interpretation that is likely to cause misperceptions. Otherwise, the expert arguably is withholding critical information from the trier of fact.

6.3   Values Placed on Avoiding False-Positive Versus False-Negative Errors

An associated practice is to select cutoffs for tests that minimize false-positive classifications but lead to relatively high false-negative error rates. Again, the expert might select a very high threshold for identifying malingering, which produces few false-positive errors but possibly frequent false-negative errors. We question whether it is proper for *experts* to tip the balance *either way*, especially without disclosing these practices, because it tends to usurp the jurors' moral or decision-making responsibilities and surreptitiously substitutes the expert's personal values. (Arguably, the situation can be different in a clinical context, where there are often strong grounds to be very conservative about identifying malingering. In clinical settings, false-positive errors may cause considerably more harm than false-negative errors, and the moral obligation is to help the patient and, above all, cause no harm.) Once more, it might be best to report the outcomes of tests and procedures explicitly and then provide interpretations. Additionally, in forensic contexts, which error is worse is not necessarily obvious or can vary. Suppose a conservative interpretive strategy leads one to misidentify a criminal who plans to kill upon release as compliant with testing and as having a psychotic disorder. If this conclusion ultimately influences institutional transfer or release, should we necessarily view the intent to minimize false-positive errors at the cost of markedly inflating the false-negative error rate as prosocial or morally compelling?

6.4   Effort Is Not All or None

Overly general descriptions are sometimes too readily assigned to outcomes on effort tests. A person who does not exceed cutoffs designed to identify *poor* effort on a measure or two has not necessarily put forth *good* effort across the evaluative session. Alternatively, a brain-injured patient with limited endurance who is given a malingering measure a couple of hours into the testing session and obtains a depressed score may have exerted excellent effort for about the first hour and modest effort for some period beyond that. The first author is aware of legal cases in which plaintiffs were said to have made poor effort and yet, on a variety of neuropsychological measures, performed at levels comparable to preaccident testing.

Although posing practical difficulties, the recommendation has sometimes been made to intersperse measures of effort across evaluation sessions (e.g., Heilbronner et al., 2009), which could help to discourage overly global judgments. Moreover, in many circumstances, we lack the required scientific knowledge to determine the extent of generalization from low performance on an effort test to performance on various tests of ability. A poor result on a measure of effort may place results on other tests in question but of course will not establish unequivocally that they underrepresent ability or especially that functioning is intact. For example, a person who underperforms might also be injured or impaired. As we have emphasized throughout the volume, these messier or more complex presentations remain less well understood and need to be investigated much more extensively.

6.5 Extreme Results of Malingering Tests Are Often Not What They Seem

Due to flaws in research designs or sampling methods, some malingering tests generate absurdly extreme results (e.g., Mr. Smith's score falls 7.4 SD below the mean for an injured group). In a normal distribution, a z score of -5.0 occurs in less than 1 per 3,000,000 individuals, of -6.0 in less than 1 per 1,000,000,000 individuals, and a score of -7.0 is infinitesimally small. Although various malingering tests do show strong features and are welcome additions to the field, these sorts of z scores should not be taken seriously because they are usually produced by skewed or distorted distributions and other methodological artifacts. As we have also described at length, due to the EGP, research often produces inflated accuracy rates or effect sizes. The concern is that these inflated results may be interpreted or presented literally, creating a gross misimpression about the strength of the evidence or the surety with which malingering has been detected. Such practices represent a potential gross injustice to the litigant and arguably should be flagged and strongly discouraged by the profession.

6.6 Response Set Measures on Questionnaires/Appraisal Of Informants

Unlike measures of ability, on which individuals cannot intentionally perform better than they are able, faking good or dissimulation can occur on the ever growing range of questionnaires used in clinical and forensic evaluations in neuropsychology. The development of questionnaires to measure such domains as everyday capacities and executive functions seeks to fill important gaps within the field and can add important information to assessments. This is not an appropriate forum to address the strengths and weakness of such questionnaires comprehensively. We would simply note that subscales within questionnaires that are designed to detect over- or underreporting often have not been adequately studied. There seems to be a tendency at times to accept results on such response set measures almost at face value or by default, even if there is little or no research on the topic. Accurate measurement of response set can be demanding, and it may take extensive effort to evaluate, refine, and modify scales to reach modest or greater levels of validity. To assume such a positive accomplishment has been realized without scientific testing or on the basis of an isolated study or two can be wishful thinking. Additionally, for more traditional personality tests that are used in the context of neuropsychological evaluation, with the exception of the MMPI-2, the available literature on response sets is often inadequate or has generated mixed outcomes (see Rogers, 2008).

When conducting forensic assessments, it is often wise to seek information from collateral sources. Information gathering may involve interviews, the use of third-party (other) reporting forms that are available for various questionnaires, or both. It would seem prudent to use at least one method that provides a check on reporting tendencies, although again scientific foundations for assessing response set may be weak or practically nonexistent. Additional research and refinement of response set measures both for self-report and third-party versions of questionnaires and various personality tests used in neuropsychology would facilitate forensic evaluation. Furthermore, even if assessment methods are limited to interview, continuing efforts to develop structured procedures specifically aimed at neuropsychological issues (e.g., post-concussion symptoms) and which include appraisal of response sets could be very valuable.

6.7   Potential Benefits of Adaptive Testing

Increased efforts to explore the use of adaptive testing in malingering assessment (and neuropsychology in general) might prove fruitful. Adaptive testing offers the advantages of flexibility while potentially maintaining the types of formalization and scientific grounding that bolster decision accuracy. None of the authors doubt the potential value of flexibility or modification of procedures in relation to the questions at hand and initial testing results. Rather, the primary concern is with the methodology used to implement such an approach, which is often impressionistic or overly subjective and prone to various sources of judgment error.

For example, it would be interesting to sample self-reports of intact and impaired areas of functioning and, on that basis, determine the areas in which to perform forced-choice testing. Forced-choice techniques are highly malleable and can be designed for almost any content area, and thus fitting complaints with forced-choice procedures is feasible. A study might involve random assignment of content areas for forced-choice procedures, standardized content areas, and tailored content areas in relation to self-reports of functioning. Another approach would be to briefly sample impressions of test difficulty, look for discrepancies between impressions and true difficulty, and emphasize those areas in malingering assessment. A third approach would involve tailoring malingering assessment to areas of poor performance on standard neuropsychological tests, because it is here that the question of true versus feigned deficit often becomes most relevant.

6.8   Creative Use of Simulation Designs

Simulation studies often become less valuable over time as research knowledge advances. However, simulation designs offer a number of advantages, in particular knowledge of true status and much greater control over level of effort and other variables. Given these advantages, variations on simulation designs might provide unique information, although in most cases such research falls mainly within the context of discovery and requires considerable further study to achieve verification. To provide a few examples of possible research directions, attempts could be made to appraise malingering skills and the ability to escape detection. One could then examine group differences to try to develop something akin to the MMPI-2 K scale. For example, a group that can beat one or more malingering tests or fool clinicians may show other systematic differences (e.g., suppressed variation in test scores) compared to less successful malingerers or a group with true injury.

In simulation designs, one can also systematically manipulate degrees of effort across multiple levels, such as very high, to moderately high, to moderately low, to very low. Given greater variation in levels of effort, certain trends might appear that would otherwise be missed. Within-group designs might also prove informative. Although in many cases research on a new measure starts with simulation studies, it might be interesting to reverse the order at times and use simulation designs as consistency tests. For example, suppose based on retrospective case analysis or a contrasting group method that certain performance characteristics or signs are believed to indicate the joint presence of malingering and injury. One could follow up such work with simulation designs to see if the same findings hold. Of course, although consistency or inconsistency is far from definitive, in many areas of science a fundamental validation strategy is to look for consistency in outcome across different methods for testing hypotheses or investigating phenomena.

6.9   Some Additional Thoughts on Research

Some approaches that seem promising for malingering detection represent an attempt to take commonsense considerations that many practitioners already apply impressionistically and place them on a more explicit, systematic, and formal basis to facilitate scientific testing and comparison. Ideally, the aim should be as much to verify adequate or good effort as it is to identify insufficient or poor effort.

Some disorders would seem to have relatively predictable outcomes. For example, with mild head injury, we would not expect catastrophic symptoms or a 6-month delay in symptom onset, and we would be much more likely to see problems in new learning rather than difficulties remembering major life events that occurred pre-injury. If we could develop better measures of prototypical outcome and range of expected variation from prototypicality among those with genuine disorder, and if the level of variation was not too great, we would be in much better position to say that some outcome does not fall within expectations or is not plausible. Such measurements should be reducible to one or a few dimensions, with studies conducted to look at distributions among those with and without the disorder (including those feigning). One might call these types of measures prototypicality indices. If outcome was so varied that most anything was about equally possible, it would serve as a more general warning about formulating causal judgments. A few words of caution are necessary here. We should be very careful about measures of severity, because one does not want to systematically identify those with genuine but atypically bad outcomes as malingerers. Also, failure to fit expectations for a particular type of injury only suggests that individuals do not have that type of injury, not necessarily that they are malingering—it may just be something else that ails them.

Some intentional symptom production requires constant attention. A patient who portrays a severe tremor may have difficulty doing so when fencing with the attorney on cross-examination. Using analogous approaches, we can examine what happens to intentionally produced symptoms under distracting conditions.

It may be possible to get at the intentionality of misrepresentations if we could create some index that compares the expected odds of misrepresentations working for or against the individual's self-interests and the examinee's obtained distribution. Some examinees misrepresent matters in a way that could cost them large settlement dollars. For example, some seriously impaired individuals deny problems, even when they have much to gain from accurate reporting. Other individuals show a very different pattern. For example, when it comes to remembering pre-injury events, they seem to systematically forget most of their shortcomings but remember many of their strengths; the pattern is reversed when it comes to post-injury events, in which case they show remarkable recall of their shortcomings but seem to forget most of their accomplishments. Unintentional misrepresentations are not likely to work systematically in the direction of serving the person's legal case or self-interests. It would not seem that difficult a matter to derive methods for grading level of self-interest and classifying responses. Approaches that indicate deviation from expected patterns of error might be similarly useful in identifying when individuals have underrepresented their post-event problems in a manner that could greatly impede fair resolution of their case.

A related index might measure negative consequences or events that have accrued for a person in proportion to the negative consequences claimed. Take an individual, for example, who reports intolerable pain but will not take a medication with mild side effects. One would expect some correlation between the level of suffering someone is experiencing and the level of suffering or inconvenience someone will tolerate in an effort to try to improve her lot. The examinee who claims to be deeply distressed by being off the job but will not participate in a work-hardening program or even send out applications, has experienced no loss of income as a result of a generous benefit package, and has maintained an active recreational life, would seem much more likely to be a malingerer than the individual who has voluntarily undergone multiple painful operations, has had his house repossessed, and almost never goes out with friends. This type of index bears some resemblance to comparisons between subjective complaints and hard examination findings, although it is obviously problematic that some serious physical disorders or conditions often cannot be detected objectively. Therefore, it might be helpful to examine the relation between claimed distress and the level of negative consequences that have occurred or to which the individual has submitted, such as reduction in income, pleasurable activities, and personal freedoms, and exposure to painful or dangerous medical procedures. Such indices might also consider what individuals have to gain if their legal cases are concluded in their favor.

In some situations, it is to an individual's advantage to be (or appear to be) impaired, and in other (most) instances it is advantageous to be unimpaired. For example, if an individual is feigning paralysis of a limb to obtain a large settlement, a burning building can suddenly alter the contingencies. In the course of assessment, treatment, and day-to-day living, the relative balance of incentive and disincentive for competence and impairment can shift dramatically, and in some circumstances individuals who have something to gain by being competent may not realize that their behavior could be detected or that they are falling out of role. Thus, the patient feigning neurological deficit suddenly becomes capable when appearing in a separate custody dispute, or an individual with severe spatial deficits suddenly regains abilities when taking a driving exam. Other times matters are perhaps less obvious. The patient with supposed problems in word finding becomes articulate when needing to defend herself during cross-examination, or the individual who appears to struggle with the motoric aspects of writing signs the release form for the office secretary with good quality penmanship. It seems worthwhile to try to identify instances in which the contingencies for proficiency shift and to examine the extent to which levels of performance shifts accordingly. Of course, as with other suggested indicators, the point is not merely to identify malingering but equally so to verify cooperation or lack of malingering.

The further development of procedures for assessing positive effort would be useful. One approach would be to obtain the best possible indicators of prior functioning, ideally in areas unlikely to be affected by the condition of interest and, even better, in areas that malingerers are likely to believe ought to be affected. One also would prefer measures of prior ability that were obtained in situations in which individuals would likely be motivated to do their best (e.g., pre-employment ability testing). Based on these indicators, such as scores on past aptitude testing, one can predict level of performance. When these predictions are met or exceeded, one would have potentially strong evidence of adequate effort. As a simplified example, if someone who had obtained a Full Scale IQ score of 100 on a pre-injury administration of one of the Wechsler Intelligence Scales achieved a comparable score on post-injury testing, we would have good reason to assume that adequate effort was made on the test. Decreased scores are ambiguous, but the point of this procedure is not necessarily to identify inadequate effort, because we already have methods to do that, but rather to identify good effort.

Past indicators of ability, even those unlikely to be altered by the condition at issue, are fallible indicators of post-injury abilities. The trick is to combine multiple fallible indicators properly (empirically and statistically) to construct stronger composites and to make predictions across a range of functions. One should be able to formulate error terms or distributions of expected results. We could then examine the match between expected and obtained results. For example, we might make predictions in five domains that should be unaltered by, say, mild to moderate head injury, and then look at the correspondence between the distribution of expected performance levels and that of obtained performances. In some cases at least, we might be able to obtain powerful evidence of good effort. These methods might well turn out to have excellent valid-positive rates, giving us something roughly equivalent to symptom validity testing in the domain of good effort, that is, a procedure that more often than not yields evidence of limited use (related to low sensitivity), but one in which the value of the exceptions makes it well worthwhile.

We realize that a number of issues would need to be addressed (e.g., identifying the best predictors of later performance, difficulties interpreting performance that is lower than expected, identifying areas that are unlikely to be affected by injury), but we do not see these problems as insurmountable. The potential utility that measures of good effort would have for legal and non-legal assessment would seem to warrant the attempt.

Acknowledgment The authors wish to offer their most sincere thanks to Arthur M. Horton for his remarkable patience, unfailing support for this work, and generously granting us the needed space to set out our ideas in detail. We truly appreciate it. Likewise, the authors wish to express their deepest appreciation to Cecil R. Reynolds, a steadfast and enduring supporter of our work. To be regarded favorably by one we esteem so highly is a true blessing.

References

Ægisdóttir, S., White, M. J., Spengler, P. M., Maugherman, A. S., Anderson, L. A., Cook, R. S., et al. (2006). The meta-analysis of clinical judgment project: Fifty-six years of accumulated research on clinical versus statistical prediction. *The Counseling Psychologist, 34*, 341–382.

Ahern, D. C. (2010). *Extreme group comparisons: Nature, prevalence, and impact on psychological research*. Unpublished doctoral dissertation. University of Rhode Island, Kingston, RI.

American Psychiatric Association. (2013). *Diagnostic and statistical manual of mental disorders* (5th ed.). Washington, DC: Author.

Ardila, A. (2005). Cultural values underlying psychometric cognitive testing. *Neuropsychology Review, 15*, 185–195.

Ardila, A. (2007). The impact of culture on neuropsychological test performance. In B. P. Uzzell, M. O. Pontón, & A. Ardila (Eds.), *International handbook of cross-cultural neuropsychology* (pp. 23–44). Mahwah, NJ: Erlbaum.

Arkes, H. R. (1981). Impediments to accurate clinical judgment and possible ways to minimize their impact. *Journal of Consulting and Clinical Psychology, 49*, 323–330.

Arkes, H. R., Dawes, R. M., & Christensen, C. (1986). Factors influencing the use of a decision rule in a probabilistic task. *Behavior and Human Decision Processes, 37*, 93–110.

Arkes, H. R., & Harkness, A. R. (1980). Effect of making a diagnosis on subsequent recognition of symptoms. *Journal of Experimental Psychology, 6*, 568–575.

Armstrong, J. S. (2001). Judgmental bootstrapping: Inferring experts = rules for forecasting. In J. S. Armstrong (Ed.), *Principles of forecasting: A handbook for researchers and practitioners* (pp. 171–192). Norwell, MA: Kluwer Academic Publishers.

Baade, L. E., & Schoenberg, M. R. (2004). A proposed method to estimate premorbid intelligence utilizing group achievement measures from school records. *Archives of Clinical Neuropsychology, 19*, 227–243.

Bain, K. M., Soble, J. R., Webber, T. A., Messerly, J. M., Bailey, K. C., Kirton, J. W., et al. (2019). Cross-validation of three Advanced Clinical Solutions performance validity tests: Examining combinations of measures to maximize classification of invalid performance. *Applied Neuropsychology: Adult.* https://doi.org/10.1080/23279095.2019.1585352.

Bashem, J. R., Rapport, L. J., Miller, J. B., Hanks, R. A., Axelrod, B. N., & Millis, S. R. (2014). Comparisons of five performance validity indices in bona fide and simulated traumatic brain injury. *The Clinical Neuropsychologist, 28*, 851–875.

Bauer, L., & McCaffrey, R. J. (2006). Coverage of the Test of Memory Malingering, Victoria Symptom Validity Test, and Word Memory Test on the Internet: Is test security threatened? *Archives of Clinical Neuropsychology, 21*, 121–126.

Berthelson, L., Mulchan, S. S., Odland, A. P., Miller, L. J., & Mittenberg, W. (2013). False positive diagnosis of malingering due to the use of multiple effort tests. *Brain Injury, 27*, 909–916.

Bilder, R. M., Sugar, C. A., & Helleman, G. S. (2014). Cumulative false positive rates given multiple performance validity tests: Commentary on Davis and Millis (2014) and Larrabee (2014). *The Clinical Neuropsychologist, 28*, 1212–1223.

Binder, L. M., Iverson, G. L., & Brooks, B. L. (2009). To err is human: "Abnormal" neuropsychological scores and variability are common in healthy adults. *Archives of Clinical Neuropsychology, 24*, 31–46.

Binder, L. M., & Rohling, M. L. (1996). Money matters: A meta-analytic review of the effects of financial incentives on recovery after closed-head injury. *American Journal of Psychiatry, 153*, 7–10.

Boone, K. B., Victor, T. L., Wen, J., Razani, J., & Ponton, M. (2007). The association between neuropsychological scores and ethnicity, language, and acculturation variables in a large patient population. *Archives of Clinical Neuropsychology, 22*, 355–365.

Brennan, A. M., Meyer, S., David, E., Pella, R., Hill, B. D., & Gouvier, W. D. (2009). The vulnerability to coaching across measures of effort. *The Clinical Neuropsychologist, 23*, 314–328.

Bridges, A. J., & Ahern, D. C. (2016). Assessment of malingering in minority populations. In F. R. Ferraro (Ed.), *Minority and cross-cultural aspects of neuropsychological assessment: Enduring and emerging trends* (2nd ed.). New York, NY: Taylor & Francis.

Bridges, A. J., Faust, D., & Ahern, D. C. (2009). Methods for the evaluation of sexually abused children: Reframing the clinician's task and recognizing its disparity with research on indicators. In K. Kuehnle & M. Connell (Eds.), *The evaluation of child sexual abuse allegations* (pp. 21–47). Hoboken, NJ: Wiley.

Bridgman, P. W. (1927). *The logic of modern physics.* New York: Macmillian.

Brini, S., Sohrabi, H. R., Hebert, J. J., Forrest, M. R. L., Laine, M., Hämäläinen, H., et al. (2020). Bilingualism is associated with a delayed onset of dementia but not with a lower risk of developing it: A systematic review with meta-analyses. *Neuropsychology Review, 30*, 1–24.

Brooks, B. L., Iverson, G. L., Sherman, E. M. S., & Holdnack, J. A. (2009). Healthy children and adolescents obtain some low scores across a battery of memory tests. *Journal of the International Neuropsychological Society, 15*, 613–617.

Brooks, B. L., Strauss, E., Sherman, E. M. S., Iverson, G. L., & Slick, D. J. (2009). Developments in neuropsychological assessment: Refining psychometric and clinical interpretive methods. *Canadian Psychology, 50*, 196–209.

Bush, S. S., Ruff, R. M., Tröster, A. I., Barth, J. T., Koffler, S. P., Pliskin, N. H., et al. (2005). Symptom validity assessment: Practice issues and medical necessity NAN policy and planning committee. *Archives of Clinical Neuropsychology, 20*, 419–426.

Butcher, J. N., Graham, J. R., Ben-Porath, Y. S., Tellegen, A., Dahlstrom, W. G., & Kaemmer, B. (2001). *MMPI-2 (Minnesota Multiphasic Personality Inventory-2): Manual for administration, scoring, and interpretation* (revised edition). Minneapolis: University of Minnesota Press.

Byrd, D. A., Miller, S. W., Reilly, J., Weber, S., Wall, T. L., & Heaton, R. K. (2006). Early environmental factors, ethnicity, and adult cognitive test performance. *Clinical Neuropsychologist, 20*, 243–260.

Chapman, L. J., & Chapman, J. P. (1967). Genesis of popular but erroneous psychodiagnostic observations. *Journal of Abnormal Psychology, 72*, 193–204.

Chapman, L. J., & Chapman, J. P. (1969). Illusory correlation as an obstacle to the use of valid psychodiagnostic signs. *Journal of Abnormal Psychology, 74*, 271–280.

Cliffe, M. J. (1992). Symptom-validity testing of feigned sensory or memory deficits: A further elaboration for subjects who understand the rationale. *British Journal of Clinical Psychology, 31*, 207–209.

Cohen, J. (1988). *Statistical power analysis for the behavioral sciences.* San Diego, CA: Academic Press.

Cohen, J. (1992). A power primer. *Psychological Bulletin, 112*, 155–159.

Cook, N. E., Karr, J. E., Brooks, B. L., Garcia-Barrera, M. A., Holdnack, J. A., & Iverson, G. L. (2019). Multivariate base rates for the assessment of executive functioning among children and adolescents. *Child Neuropsychology, 25*, 836–858.

Cronbach, L. J., & Meehl, P. E. (1955). Construct validity in psychological tests. *Psychological Bulletin, 52*, 281–302.

Crowe, M., Clay, O. J., Sawyer, P., Crowther, M. R., & Allman, R. M. (2008). Education and reading ability in relation to differences in cognitive screening between African American and Caucasian older adults. *International Journal of Geriatric Psychiatry, 23*, 222–223.

Davis, J. J., & Millis, S. R. (2014). Examination of performance validity test failure in relation to number of tests administered. *The Clinical Neuropsychologist, 28*, 199–214.

Dawes, R. M. (1979). The robust beauty of improper linear models in decision making. *American Psychologist, 34*, 571–582.

Dawes, R. M. (1989). Experience and validity of clinical judgment: The illusory correlation. *Behavioral Sciences & the Law, 7*, 457–467.

Dawes, R. M., Faust, D., & Meehl, P. E. (1989). Clinical versus actuarial judgment. *Science, 243*, 1668–1674.

Dawes, R. M., & Meehl, P. E. (1966). Mixed group validation: A method for determining the validity of diagnostic signs without using criterion groups. *Psychological Bulletin, 66*, 63–67.

Dean, A. C., Boone, K. B., Kim, M. S., Curiel, A. R., Martin, D. J., Victor, T. L., et al. (2008). Examination of the impact of ethnicity on the Minnesota Multiphasic Personality Inventory-2 (MMPI-2) Fake Bad Scale. *Clinical Neuropsychologist, 22*, 1054–1060.

Dumont, R., & Willis, J. O. (1995). Intrasubtest scatter on the WISC-III for various clinical samples vs. the standardization sample: An examination of WISC folklore. *Journal of Psychoeducational Assessment, 13*, 271–285.

Einhorn, H. J. (1986). Accepting error to make less error. *Journal of Personality Assessment, 50(3)*, 387–395.

Elkovitch, N., Viljoen, J. L., Scalora, M. J., & Ullman, D. (2008). Research report: Assessing risk of reoffending in adolescents who have committed a sexual offense: The accuracy of clinical judgments after completion of risk assessment instruments. *Behavioral Sciences & the Law, 26*, 511–528.

Erdodi, L. A. (2019). Aggregating validity indicators: The salience of domain specificity and the indeterminate range in multivariate models of performance validity. *Applied Neuropsychology: Adult, 26*, 155–172.

Erdodi, L. A., & Abeare, C. A. (2019). Stronger together: The Wechsler Adult Intelligence Scale—Fourth Edition as a multivariate performance validity test in patients with traumatic brain injury. *Archives of Clinical Neuropsychology, 35*, 188–204.

Fargo, J. D., Schefft, B. K., Szaflarski, J. P., Howe, S. R., Yeh, H., & Privitera, M. D. (2008). Accuracy of clinical neuropsychological versus statistical prediction in the classification of seizure types. *The Clinical Neuropsychologist, 22*, 181–194.

Faust, D. (1984). *The limits of scientific reasoning.* Minneapolis: University of Minnesota Press.

Faust, D. (1989). Data integration in legal evaluations. Can clinicians deliver on their premises? *Behavioral Sciences & the Law, 7*, 469–483.

Faust, D. (1993). The use of traditional neuropsychological tests to describe and prescribe: Why polishing the crystal ball won't help. In G. L. Glueckauf, L. B. Sechrest, G. R. Bond, & E. C. McDonel (Eds.), *Improving assessment in rehabilitation and health* (pp. 87–108). Newbury Park, CA: Sage.

Faust, D. (1997). Of science, meta-science, and clinical practice: The generalization of a generalization to a particular. *Journal of Personality Assessment, 68*, 331–354.

Faust, D. (2004). Statistical significance testing, construct validity, and clinical versus actuarial judgment: An interesting (seeming) paradox. *Applied and Preventative Psychology, 11*, 27–29.

Faust, D. (2006). Paul Meehl as methodologist-philosopher of science: the formulation of meta-science. *Journal of Abnormal Psychology, 115*, 205–209.

Faust, D. (2007). Decision research can increase the accuracy of clinical judgment and thereby improve patient care. In S. O. Lilienfeld & W. T. O'Donohue (Eds.), *The great ideas of clinical science: 17 principles that every mental health professional should understand* (pp. 49–76). New York: Routledge.

Faust, D. (2008). Why meta-science should be irresistible to decision researchers. In J. Krueger (Ed.), *Rationality and social responsibility: Essays in honor of Robyn Mason Dawes* (pp. 91–110). New York: Psychology Press.

Faust, D. (2011). *Coping with psychiatric and psychological testimony*. New York: Oxford University Press.

Faust, D., & Ackley, M. A. (1998). Did you think it was going to be easy? Some methodological suggestions for the investigation and development of malingering detection techniques. In C. R. Reynolds (Ed.), *Detection of malingering during head injury litigation* (pp. 1–54). New York: Plenum.

Faust, D., & Ahern, D. C. (2011). Clinical judgment and prediction. In D. Faust (Ed.), *Coping with psychiatric and psychological testimony* (6th ed.). New York: Oxford University Press.

Faust, D., Ahern, D. C., & Bridges, A. J. (2011). Neuropsychological (brain damage) assessment. In D. Faust (Ed.), *Coping with psychiatric and psychological testimony* (6th ed.). New York: Oxford University Press.

Faust, D., Ahern, D. C., & Bridges, A. J. (in preparation). Obstacles to complex pattern analysis in neuropsychology and more effective alternatives.

Faust, D., Bridges, A. J., & Ahern, D. C. (2009a). Methods for the evaluation of sexually abused children: Issues and needed features for abuse indicators. In K. Kuehnle & M. Connell (Eds.), *The evaluation of child sexual abuse allegations* (pp. 3–19). Hoboken, NJ: Wiley.

Faust, D., Bridges, A. J., & Ahern, D. C. (2009b). Methods for the evaluation of sexually abused children: Suggestions for clinical work and research. In K. Kuehnle & M. Connell (Eds.), *The evaluation of child sexual abuse allegations* (pp. 49–66). Hoboken, NJ: Wiley.

Faust, D., & Faust, K. (2011). Experts' experience and diagnostic and predictive accuracy. In D. Faust (Ed.), *Coping with psychiatric and psychological testimony*. New York: Oxford University Press.

Faust, D., Hart, K., & Guilmette, T. J. (1988). Pediatric malingering: The capacity of children to fake believable deficits on neuropsychological testing. *Journal of Consulting and Clinical Psychology, 56*, 578–582.

Faust, D., Hart, K., Guilmette, T. J., & Arkes, H. R. (1988). Neuropsychologists' capacity to detect adolescent malingerers. *Professional Psychology: Research and Practice, 19*, 508–515.

Faust, D., & Meehl, P. E. (1992). Using scientific methods to resolve questions in the history and philosophy of science: Some illustrations. *Behavior Therapy, 23*, 195–211.

Frederick, R. I. (2003). *Validity Indicator Profile. Manual*. Minneapolis, MN: Pearson.

Frederick, R. I., & Bowden, S. C. (2009). The test validation summary. *Assessment, 16*, 215–236.

Frederick, R. I., & Foster, H. G., Jr. (1991). Multiple measures of malingering on a forced-choice test of cognitive ability. *Psychological Assessment, 3*, 596–602.

Galanter, C. A., & Patel, V. L. (2005). Medical decision making: A selective review for child psychiatrists and psychologists. *Journal of Child Psychology and Psychiatry, 46*, 675–689.

Garb, H. N., & Schramke, C. J. (1996). Judgment research and neuropsychological assessment: A narrative review and meta-analyses. *Psychological Bulletin, 120*, 140–153.

Goldberg, L. R. (1968). Simple models or simple processes? Some research on clinical judgments. *American Psychologist, 23*, 483–496.

Goldberg, L. R. (1991). Human mind versus regression equation: Five contrasts. In D. Cicchetti & W. M. Grove (Eds.), *Thinking clearly about psychology: Essays in honor of Paul E. Meehl: Vol. 1. Matters of public interest* (pp. 173–184). Minneapolis: University of Minnesota Press.

Golden, M. (1964). Some effects of combining psychological tests on clinical inferences. *Journal of Consulting Psychology, 28*, 440–446.

Gough, H. G. (1954). Some common misconceptions about neuroticism. *Journal of Consulting Psychology, 18*, 287–292.

Gouvier, W. D. (2001). Are you sure you're really telling the truth? *NeuroRehabilitation, 16*, 215–219.

Gouvier, W. D., Cubic, B., Jones, G., Brantley, P., & Cutlip, Q. (1992). Post-concussion symptoms and daily stress in normal and head-injured college populations. *Archives of Clinical Neuropsychology, 7*, 193–211.

Gouvier, W. D., Uddo-Crane, M., & Brown, L. M. (1988). Base rates for post-concussional symptoms. *Archives of Clinical Neuropsychology, 3*, 273–278.

Greene, R. L. (2011). *The MMPI-2/MMPI-2-RF: An interpretive manual* (3rd ed.). Boston: Allyn & Bacon.

Greenwald, A. G., Pratkanis, A. R., Leippe, M. R., & Baumgardner, M. H. (1986). Under what conditions does theory obstruct research progress? *Psychological Review, 93*, 216–229.

Grove, W. M., & Lloyd, M. (2006). Meehl's contribution to clinical versus statistical prediction. *Journal of Abnormal Psychology, 115*, 192–194.

Grove, W. M., Zald, D. H., Lebow, B. S., Snitz, B. E., & Nelson, C. (2000). Clinical vs. mechanical prediction: A meta-analysis. *Psychological Assessment, 12*, 19–30.

Guilbault, R. L., Bryant, F. B., Brockway, J. H., & Posavac, E. J. (2004). A meta-analysis of research on hindsight bias. *Basic and Applied Social Psychology, 26*, 103–117.

Gunstad, J., & Suhr, J. A. (2004). Cognitive factors in Postconcussion Syndrome symptom report. *Archives of Clinical Neuropsychology, 19*, 391–404.

Hambleton, R. K., Merenda, P. F., & Spielberger, D. C. (Eds.). (2005). *Adapting educational and psychological tests for cross-cultural assessment*. Mahwah, NJ: Erlbaum.

Hanson, R. K., & Morton-Bourgon, K. E. (2009). The accuracy of recidivism risk assessments for sexual offenders: A meta-analysis of 118 prediction studies. *Psychological Assessment, 21*, 1–21.

Heaton, R. K., Ryan, L., & Grant, I. (2009). Demographic influences and use of demographically corrected norms in neuropsychological assessment. In I. Grant & K. M. Adams (Eds.), *Neuropsychological assessment of neuropsychiatric and neuromedical disorders* (pp. 127–155). New York: Oxford University Press.

Heilbronner, R. L., Sweet, J. J., Morgan, J. E., Larrabee, G. J., & Millis, S. R. (2009). American Academy of Clinical Neuropsychology Consensus Conference statement on the neuropsychological assessment of effort, response bias, and malingering. *The Clinical Neuropsychologist, 23*, 1093–1129.

Herman, S. (2005). Improving decision making in forensic child sexual abuse evaluations. *Law and Human Behavior, 29*, 87–120.

Hogarth, R. M., & Karelaia, N. (2007). Heuristic and linear models of judgment: Matching rules and environments. *Psychological Review, 114*, 733–758.

Hyman, R. (1977). "Cold reading": How to convince strangers that you know all about them. *The Zetetic, 1*, 18–37.

Iverson, G. L., & Lange, R. T. (2003). Examination of "postconcussion-like" symptoms in a healthy sample. *Applied Neuropsychology, 10*, 137–144.

Jewsbury, P. A., & Bowden, S. C. (2014). A description of mixed group validation. *Assessment, 21*, 170–180.

Kaiser Family Foundation. (2011). *Poverty rates by race/ethnicity, US (2009)*. Retrieved February 11, 2011, from http://www.statehealthfacts.org/.

Kareken, D. A., & Williams, J. M. (1994). Human judgment and estimation of premorbid intellectual function. *Psychological Assessment, 6*, 83–91.

Kennedy, M. L., Willis, W. G., & Faust, D. (1997). The base-rate fallacy in school psychology. *Journal of Psychoeducational Assessment, 15*, 292–307.

Labarge, A. S., McCaffrey, R. J., & Brown, T. A. (2003). Neuropsychologists' abilities to determine the predictive value of diagnostic tests. *Archives of Clinical Neuropsychology, 18*, 165–175.

LaDuke, C., Barr, W., Brodale, D. L., & Rabin, L. A. (2018). Toward generally accepted forensic assessment practices among clinical neuropcyhologists: A survey of professional practice and common test use. *The Clinical Neuropsychologist, 32*, 145–164.

Larrabee, G. J. (2014). False-positive rates associated with the use of multiple performance and symptoms validity tests. *Archives of Clinical Neuropsychology, 29*, 364–373.

Leli, D. A., & Filskov, S. B. (1981). Clinical-actuarial detection and description of brain impairment with the W-B form 1. *Journal of Clinical Psychology, 37*, 623–629.

Llorente, A., Soong, C., Friedrich, E., Shields, B., Cohen, P., Dias, E., et al. (2017). Neuropsychological and legal factors affecting unaccompanied immigrant children: A review of the literature and case study. *Journal of Pediatric Neuropsychology, 3*, 170–188.

Manly, J. J., & Jacobs, D. M. (2002). Future directions in neuropsychological assessment with African Americans. In F. R. Ferraro (Ed.), *Minority and cross-cultural aspects of neuropsychological assessment* (pp. 79–96). Exton, PA: Swets & Zeitlinger.

Martin, P. K., Schroeder, R. W., Olsen, D. H., Maloy, H., Boettcher, A., Ernst, N., et al. (2019). A systematic review and meta-analysis of the Test of Memory Malingering in adults: Two decades of deception detection. *The Clinical Neuropsychologist, 34*, 88–119.

Meehl, P. E. (1954/1996). *Clinical versus statistical prediction: A theoretical analysis and a review of the evidence*. Minneapolis: University of Minnesota Press. Reprinted with new Preface, 1996, by Jason Aronson, Northvale, NJ.

Meehl, P. E. (1984). *Foreword to Faust, D., The limits of scientific reasoning*. Minneapolis: University of Minnesota Press.

Meehl, P. E. (1986). Causes and effects of my disturbing little book. *Journal of Personality Assessment, 50*, 370–375.

Meehl, P. E. (1990). Why summaries of research on psychological theories are often uninterpretable. *Psychological Reports, 66*, 195–244.

Meehl, P. E. (1991). In C. A. Anderson & K. Gunderson (Eds.), *Selected philosophical and methodological papers*. Minneapolis: University of Minnesota Press.

Meehl, P. E. (1992). Needs (Murry, 1938) and state-variables (Skinner, 1938). *Psychological Reports, 70*, 407–451.

Meehl, P. E. (1995). Bootstraps taxometrics: Solving the classification problem in psychopathology. *American Psychologist, 50*, 266–275.

Meehl, P. E. (1999). Clarifications about taxometric method. *Journal of Applied and Preventive Psychology, 8*, 165–174.

Meehl, P. E. (2001). Comorbidity and taxometrics. *Clinical Psychology: Science and Practice, 8*, 507–519.

Meehl, P. E. (2004). What's in a taxon? *Journal of Abnormal Psychology, 113*, 39–43.

Meehl, P. E. (2006). In N. G. Waller, L. J. Yonce, W. M. Grove, D. Faust, & M. F. Lenzenweger (Eds.), *A Paul Meehl Reader: Essays on the practice of scientific psychology*. Mahwah, NJ: Erlbaum.

Meehl, P. E., & Rosen, A. (1955). Antecedent probability and the efficiency of psychometric signs, patterns, or cutting scores. *Psychological Bulletin, 52*, 194–216. Reprinted in N. G. Waller, L. J. Yonce, W. M. Grove, D. Faust, & M. F. Lenzenweger (Eds.), A Paul Meehl reader: Essays on the practice of scientific psychology (pp. 213–236). Mahwah, NJ: Lawrence Erlbaum, 2006.

Mittenberg, W., DiGiulio, D. V., Perrin, S., & Bass, A. E. (1992). Symptoms following mild head injury: Expectation as etiology. *Journal of Neurology, Neurosurgery, and Psychiatry, 55*, 200–204.

Nabors, N. A., Evans, J. D., & Strickland, T. L. (2000). Neuropsychological assessment and intervention with African Americans. In E. Fletcher-Janzen, T. L. Strickland, & C. R. Reynolds (Eds.), *Handbook of cross-cultural neuropsychology* (pp. 31–42). New York: Kluwer Academic/Plenum.

Neisser, U., Boodoo, G., Bouchard, T. J., Jr., Boykin, A. W., Brody, N., Ceci, S. J., et al. (1996). Intelligence: Knowns and unknowns. *American Psychologist, 51*, 77–101.

Nelson, A. (2002). Unequal treatment: Confronting racial and ethnic disparities in health care. *Journal of the National Medical Association, 94*, 666–668.

Nickerson, R. S. (1998). Confirmation bias: A ubiquitous phenomenon in many guises. *Review of General Psychology, 2*, 175–220.

Nickerson, R. S. (2004). *Cognition and chance: The psychology of probabilistic reasoning.* Mahwah, NJ: Erlbaum.

Nijdam-Jones, A., Rivera, D., Rosenfeld, B., & Arango-Lasprilla, J. C. (2019). The effect of literacy and culture on cognitive effort test performance: An examination of the Test of Memory Malingering in Colombia. *Journal of Clinical and Experimental Neuropsychology, 41*, 1015–1023.

Nijdam-Jones, A., & Rosenfeld, B. (2017). Cross-cultural feigning assessment: A systematic review of feigning instruments used with linguistically, ethnically, and culturally diverse samples. *Psychological Assessment, 29*, 1321–1336.

Orme, D., Ree, M. J., & Rioux, P. (2001). Premorbid IQ estimates from a multiple aptitude test battery: Regression vs. equating. *Archives of Clinical Neuropsychology, 16*, 679–688.

Razani, J., Burciaga, J., Madore, M., & Wong, J. (2007). Effects of acculturation on tests of attention and information processing in an ethnically diverse group. *Archives of Clinical Neuropsychology, 22*, 333–341.

Reesman, J. H., Day, L. A., Szymanski, C. A., Hughes-Wheatland, R., Witkin, G. A., Kalback, S. R., et al. (2014). Review of intellectual assessment measures for children who are deaf or hard of hearing. *Rehabilitation Psychology, 59*, 99–106.

Reichenbach, H. (1938). *Experience and prediction.* Chicago: University of Chicago Press.

Reitan, R. M., & Wolfson, D. (1993). *The Halstead–Reitan Neuropsychological Test Battery: Theory and clinical interpretation* (2nd ed.). Tucson, AZ: Neuropsychology Press.

Reynolds, C. R. (1997). Postscripts on premorbid ability estimation: Conceptual addenda and a few words on alternative and conditional approaches. *Archives of Clinical Neuropsychology, 12*, 769–778.

Reynolds, C. R. (1998). Common sense, clinicians, and actuarialism in the detection of malingering during head injury litigation. In C. R. Reynolds (Ed.), *Detection of malingering during head injury litigation* (pp. 261–286). New York: Plenum.

Rogers, R. (1990a). Development of a new classificatory model of malingering. *Bulletin of the American Academy of Psychiatry and Law, 18*, 323–333.

Rogers, R. (1990b). Models of feigned mental illness. *Professional Psychology: Research and Practice, 21*, 182–188.

Rogers, R. (Ed.). (2008). *Clinical assessment of malingering and deception* (3rd ed.). New York: Guilford.

Rogers, R., Bagby, R. M., & Chakraborty, D. (1993). Feigning schizophrenic disorders on the MMPI-2: Detection of coached simulators. *Journal of Personality Assessment, 60*, 215–226.

Rogers, R., Sewell, K. W., Martin, M. A., & Vitacco, M. J. (2003). Detection of feigned mental disorders: A meta-analysis of the MMPI-2 and malingering. *Assessment, 10*, 160–177.

Rosselli, M., & Ardila, A. (2003). The impact of culture and education on non-verbal neuropsychological measurements: A critical review. *Brain and Cognition, 52*, 326–333.

Ruscio, J. (2003). Holistic judgment in clinical practice. *The Scientific Review of Mental Health Practice, 2*, 38–48.

Salazar, X. F., Lu, P. H., Wen, J., & Boone, K. B. (2007). The use of effort tests in ethnic minorities and in non-English-speaking and English as a second language populations. In K. B. Boone (Ed.), *Assessment of feigned cognitive impairment: A neuropsychological perspective* (pp. 405–427). New York: Guilford.

Satcher, D. (2001). *Mental health: Culture, race, and ethnicity—A supplement to Mental health: A report of the Surgeon General.* Rockville, MD: U.S. Department of Health and Human Services.

Sawyer, J. (1966). Measurement and prediction, clinical and statistical. *Psychological Bulletin, 66*, 178–200.

Sbordone, R. J., Strickland, T. L., & Purisch, A. D. (2000). Neuropsychological assessment of the criminal defendant: The significance of cultural factors. In E. Fletcher-Janzen, T. L. Strickland, & C. R. Reynolds (Eds.), *Handbook of crosscultural neuropsychology* (pp. 335–344). New York: Kluwer Academic/Plenum.

Schretlen, D. J., Buffington, A. L. H., Meyer, S. M., & Pearlson, G. D. (2005). The use of word-reading to estimate "premorbid" ability in cognitive domains other than intelligence. *Journal of the International Neuropsychological Society, 11*, 784–787.

Schretlen, D. J., Munro, C. A., Anthony, J. C., & Pearlson, G. D. (2003). Examining the range of normal intraindividual variability in neuropsychological test performance. *Journal of the International Neuropsychological Society, 9*, 864–870.

Schretlen, D. J., & Sullivan, C. (2013). Intraindividual variability in cognitive test performance. In S. Koffler, J. Morgan, I. S. Baron, & M. F. Greiffenstein (Eds.), *AACN neuropsychology in review. Neuropsychology: Science and practice, 1* (pp. 39–60). New York: Oxford University Press.

Sharland, M. J., & Gfeller, J. D. (2007). A survey of neuropsychologists' beliefs and practices with respect to the assessment of effort. *Archives of Clinical Neuropsychology, 22*, 213–223.

Sieck, W. R., & Arkes, H. R. (2005). The recalcitrance of overconfidence and its contribution to decision aid neglect. *Journal of Behavioral Decision Making, 18*, 29–53.

Simon, H. A. (1956). Rational choice and the structure of environments. *Psychological Review, 63*, 129–138.

Simon, H. A. (1957). *Models of man.* New York: Wiley.

Slick, D. J., Tan, J. E., Strauss, E. H., & Hultsch, D. F. (2004). Detecting malingering: A survey of experts' practices. *Archives of Clinical Neuropsychology, 19*, 465–473.

Strong, D. R., Glassmire, D. M., Frederick, R. I., & Greene, R. L. (2006). Evaluating the latent structure of the MMPI-2 F(p) scale in a forensic sample: A taxometric analysis. *Psychological Assessment, 18*, 250–261.

Strong, D. R., Greene, R. L., & Schinka, J. A. (2000). A taxometric analysis of MMPI-2 infrequency scales [F and F(p)] in clinical settings. *Psychological Assessment, 12*, 166–173.

Tan, Y. W., Burgess, G. H., & Green, R. J. (2020). The effects of acculturation on neuropsychological test performance: A systematic literature review. *The Clinical Neuropsychologist.* https://doi.org/10.1080/13854046.2020.1714740.

Tombaugh, T. N. (1996). *Test of Memory Malingering (TOMM).* North Tonawanda, NY: Multi-Health Systems, Inc..

Tsushima, W. T., & Tsushima, V. G. (2009). Comparison of MMPI-2 validity scales among compensation-seeking Caucasian and Asian American medical patients. *Assessment, 6*, 159–164.

Vickery, C. D., Berry, D. T. R., Inman, T. H., Harris, M. J., & Orey, S. A. (2001). Detection of inadequate effort on neuropsychological testing: A meta-analytic review of selected procedures. *Archives of Clinical Neuropsychology, 16*, 45–73.

Vilar-Lopez, R., Santiago-Ramajo, S., Gomez-Rio, M., Verdejo-Garcia, A., Llamas, J. M., & Perez-Garcia, M. (2007). Detection of malingering in a Spanish population using three specific malingering tests. *Archives of Clinical Psychology, 22*, 379–388.

Waller, N. G., & Meehl, P. E. (1998). *Multivariate taxometric procedures: Distinguishing types from continua.* Thousand Oaks, CA: Sage.

Waller, N. G., Yonce, L. J., Grove, W. M., Faust, D., & Lenzenweger, M. F. (Eds.). (2006). *A Paul Meehl reader: Essays on the practice of scientific psychology*. Mahwah, NJ: Lawrence Erlbaum.

Walters, G. D., Berry, D. T. R., Rogers, R., Payne, J. M., & Granacher, R. P., Jr. (2009). Feigned neurocognitive deficit: Taxon or dimension? *Journal of Clinical and Experimental Neuropsychology, 31*, 584–593.

Walters, G. D., Rogers, R., Berry, D. T. R., Miller, H. A., Duncan, S. A., McCusker, P. J., et al. (2008). Malingering as a categorical or dimensional construct: The latent structure of feigned psychopathology as measured by the SIRS and MMPI-2. *Psychological Assessment, 20*, 238–247.

Watkins, M. W., Glutting, J. J., & Youngstrom, E. A. (2005). Issues in subtest profile analysis. In D. P. Flanagan & P. L. Harrison (Eds.), *Contemporary intellectual assessment: Theories, tests, and issues* (pp. 251–268). New York: Guilford.

Wechsler, D. (2008). *Wechsler Adult Intelligence Scale, Fourth Edition: Administration and scoring manual*. San Antonio, TX: The Psychological Corporation.

Wedding, D. (1983). Clinical and statistical prediction in neuropsychology. *Clinical Neuropsychology, 5*, 49–55.

Wedding, D., & Faust, D. (1989). Clinical judgment and decision making in neuropsychology. *Archives of Clinical Neuropsychology, 4*, 233–265.

Wetter, M. W., Baer, R. A., Berry, D. T. R., & Reynolds, S. K. (1994). The effect of symptom information on faking on the MMI-2. *Assessment, 1*, 199–207.

Williams, J. M. (1997). The prediction of premorbid memory ability. *Archives of Clinical Neuropsychology, 12*, 745–756.

Williams, J. M. (1998). The malingering of memory disorder. In C. R. Reynolds (Ed.), *Detection of malingering during head injury litigation* (pp. 105–132). New York: Plenum.

Wong, J. L., Regennitter, R. P., & Barris, F. (1994). Base rates and simulated symptoms of mild head injury among normals. *Archives of Clinical Neuropsychology, 9*, 411–425.

Yager, J. (1977). Psychiatric eclecticism: A cognitive view. *American Journal of Psychiatry, 134*, 736–741.

Printed by Printforce, the Netherlands